Managing Children with Psychiatric Problems

Second edition

Managing Children with Psychiatric Problems

Second edition

Edited by

M Elena Garralda

Academic Unit of Child and Adolescent Psychiatry, Imperial College, London, UK

Caroline Hyde

Consultant Child and Adolescent Psychiatrist, Thelma Golding Centre, Hounslow, UK

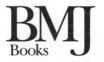

First published in 1993
Second edition 2003
by BMJ Books, BMA House, Tavistock Square,
London WC1H 9JR

www.bmjbooks.com

British Library Cataloguing in Publication Data

A catalogue record for this book is available from the British Library

ISBN 0 7279 1567 3

Typeset by SIVA Math Setters, Chennai, India
Printed and bound in Spain by Graphycems, Navarra

Contents

Sadly Dr Bridget O'Shea died after writing her contribution to this book.

Contributors

Veira Bailey
Consultant Child and Adolescent Psychiatrist, Knightsbridge, London, UK

Harold Behr
Consultant Child and Adolescent Psychiatrist, North London Centre for Group Therapy, London, UK

Eric Fombonne
Canada Research Chair in Child Psychiatry, Professor of Psychiatry, McGill University, and Director of the Department of Psychiatry, Montreal Children's Hospital, Montreal, Canada

Gillian C Forrest
Consultant Child Psychiatrist and Honorary Senior Lecturer, Park Hospital for Children, Oxford, UK

David Goldberg
Consultant Adolescent Psychiatrist, Adolescent Service, Wandsworth, South West London and St George's Mental Health Trust, London, UK

Philip Graham
Emeritus Professor of Child Psychiatry, Institute of Child Health, London, UK

Richard Harrington
Professor in the Department of Child and Adolescent Psychiatry, Royal Manchester Children's Hospital, Manchester, UK

Matthew Hodes
Senior Lecturer in Child and Adolescent Psychiatry, Academic Unit of Child and Adolescent Psychiatry, Imperial College, London, UK

Bridget O'Shea
Late Consultant Child and Adolescent Psychiatrist, Thelma Golding Centre, Hounslow, UK

John Pearce
Professor Emeritus of Child and Adolescent Psychiatry, University of Nottingham, Nottingham, UK

Michael Prendergast
Consultant Child and Teenage Psychiatrist, Prudhoe Hospital, Prudhoe, UK

Stephen Scott
Reader in Child Health and Behaviour, and Consultant Child and Adolescent Psychiatrist, Institute of Psychiatry and Maudsley Hospital, London, UK

Michael Shaw
Consultant Child Psychiatrist, Cotswold House, Sutton, Surrey, UK

Claire Sturge
Consultant Child and Adolescent Psychiatrist, Gayton Child and Family Centre, Harrow, UK

Margaret JJ Thompson
Senior Clinical Lecturer/Consultant Child and Adolescent Psychiatrist, Child and Adolescent Mental Health Services, Child and Family Health Centre, The Ashurst Centre, Southampton, UK

Judith Trowell
Consultant Child and Adolescent Psychiatrist, Tavistock Clinic, London and Honorary Senior Lecturer, Royal Free and UCL Medical School, London

Bea Vickers
Consultant Child and Adolescent Psychiatrist, South West London and St George's Mental Health NHS Trust, London, UK

Preface

The popularity of the first edition of this book together with clear changes in child psychiatric practice over the past 10 years have led to this second edition. The aim is still, as outlined in the preface to the first edition, to provide readable accounts of the rationale and reality of child and adolescent psychiatric work by experienced practitioners in the field. We have made changes to the topics covered to reflect the increasingly evidence-based nature of child and adolescent psychiatric practice: chapters on cognitive and interpersonal therapies are now included under specific types of treatment, under liaison with other services there are now chapters on working with primary care and educational services; and a contribution on legal aspects has also been added. We hope that this new edition will help paediatricians, general practitioners, and other doctors and professionals working with children to address the psychiatric aspects of their practice.

Elena Garralda, Caroline Hyde

Section I
Overview

1: Identifying psychiatric disorders in children

JOHN PEARCE

Overview

Psychiatric disorders in children may present as anomalous behaviour, emotions and/or thought processes.

Identification of mental health problems in children is a complex process, taking into consideration the duration, frequency and severity of the problem, and the child's stage of development.

The assessment must take the following factors into account: individual factors that predispose young people to mental health problems, including family, school, and peer influences, protective factors.

Introduction

Children who have a psychiatric disorder are often seen as being difficult rather than disturbed, and the significance of the emotion or the behaviour may easily be missed. The distinction between "normal" and pathological behaviour is important because reassurance is appropriate in the first case and dangerous in the latter.

A psychiatric disorder can be classified as anomalous behaviour, emotions, or thought processes (the three main aspects of mental functioning) that are so prolonged or severe, or both, that they interfere with everyday life and are a handicap to the child or those who care for the child. The child's stage of development and the sociocultural context in which the disorder occurs must also be taken into account (Box 1.1).

Box 1.1 Definition of childhood psychiatric disorder

Anomalies in the child's behaviour, emotion, or thoughts
Persistent – for at least two weeks
Severe enough to interfere with the child's everyday life
A handicap to the child or their carers, or both
Taking account of the child's stage of development
Taking account of the sociocultural context.

Rarely, a child's mental state may lead to behaviour so bizarre or extreme that it only has to occur once to be regarded as abnormal.

Psychiatric disorder in children, as defined above, has a one year prevalence of roughly 10% in the general population, which is much the same as that in adults. This rate is influenced by several risk and protective factors.

Risk factors for psychiatric disorders in children

Child risk factors

Surveillance for psychiatric disorder is assisted by a knowledge of the main factors that increase risk. The most important intrinsic or child based influences that put a child at risk are given in Box 1.2. Most children with psychiatric disorder will have been unfavourably influenced by more than just a single risk factor. Each of the risk factors interacts with others in such a way that the total adversity is more than the sum of the individual factors. Thus, a 10 year old boy with epilepsy and learning difficulties may have no problems until he is teased for being slow at school, which results in low self esteem, and that in turn interferes with his motivation to learn.

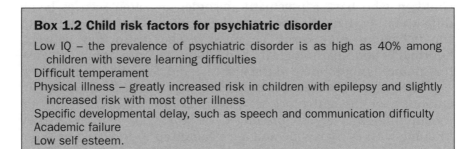

Box 1.2 Child risk factors for psychiatric disorder

Low IQ – the prevalence of psychiatric disorder is as high as 40% among children with severe learning difficulties
Difficult temperament
Physical illness – greatly increased risk in children with epilepsy and slightly increased risk with most other illness
Specific developmental delay, such as speech and communication difficulty
Academic failure
Low self esteem.

The cumulative effect of stress can have a potent negative influence on children. Children who have experienced more than two adverse life events in the recent past are particularly susceptible to developing emotional or behavioural problems. There is evidence that some life stress factors may lie dormant for many years (the sleeper effect) only to have an effect when "awoken" by a related adverse experience. This increased vulnerability to stress may be seen in the abnormal behaviour of some teenagers who have been sexually abused or subjected to other detrimental influences much earlier in their childhood.

Boys are generally more prone to development of psychiatric disorder, much as they are more vulnerable to almost every life adversity. The difference in the rates of psychiatric disorders in girls and boys tends to be less pronounced in preschool children. During adolescence, however, girls become more vulnerable, mainly because they have higher rates of emotional disorder. Throughout childhood boys are more likely to experience developmental disorders, behaviour problems, and conduct disorder.

Family and other external risk factors

Family risk factors are especially complex because there are many possible interactions (Box 1.3). Family breakdown is a good example of a process of adverse events and interactions that multiply the risk of psychopathology. Thus, children from a broken home may copy the parental model of unsatisfactory relationships and poor communication, and become increasingly difficult to manage. The child's behaviour is then likely to lead to critical and hostile parental responses that only serve to make the child more disturbed. This results in a prevalence of psychiatric disorder as high as 80% during the first year after divorce. The rate of childhood psychiatric disorder is also raised before and for many years after parental separation. This contrasts with the loss of a parent by death, which gives only a slightly increased risk of psychiatric disorder.

Box 1.3 Family factors that increase the risk of psychiatric disorder

Family breakdown
Maternal mental ill health
Paternal criminality, alcoholism, or psychopathy
Abuse
Poverty, whatever the cause
Overt parental conflict
Inconsistent, unclear, or critical discipline
Hostile and rejecting relationships
Failure to adapt to the child's developmental needs
Death and loss, including loss of friendships.

Maternal, but not paternal, mental illness increases the risk of psychiatric disorder. A child's vulnerability to a depressed mother may be increased during critical periods of development, for example during the time when the mother is bonding to the child in the first few weeks after birth. There is also evidence that some children continue to have problems even after the mother's depression has resolved, suggesting that a process of negative behaviour has been established that becomes difficult to disentangle. Very young children are strongly influenced by the mood of their parents, but as they grow

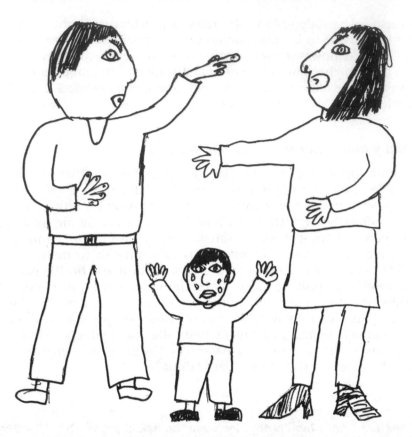

"My parents don't get on." Sometimes, children's disturbance is closely related to family problems

older other factors such as school, peers, and culture have a more powerful effect. Children spend a minimum of some 15 000 hours in school. It is therefore no surprise to find that experiences at school, such as bullying, school organisation, and academic achievement, can influence the rate of childhood psychiatric disorder (Box 1.4).

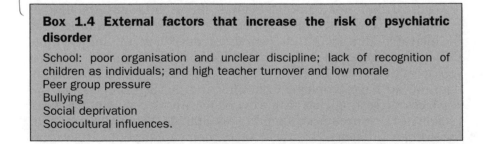

Box 1.4 External factors that increase the risk of psychiatric disorder

School: poor organisation and unclear discipline; lack of recognition of children as individuals; and high teacher turnover and low morale
Peer group pressure
Bullying
Social deprivation
Sociocultural influences.

Protective factors against psychiatric disorders in children

The risk factors outlined above are common to many children and yet only a minority at any one time actually suffer from a formal psychiatric disorder. So why do some children cope well and not develop a psychiatric disorder, even though they have many adversities stacked up against them? One of the most powerful protective factors of all is positive self esteem. Self image develops slowly and becomes relatively fixed by age 7–8 years. It is crucially dependent on how parents and others have responded to the child. The presence of an affectionate and trusting relationship with an adult is therefore also protective. A stable temperament and a good level of intelligence will help a child to adapt to stressful situations and reduce the risk of psychiatric disorder (Box 1.5).

Box 1.5 Factors that protect against psychiatric disorder

Positive self image
Affectionate relationships
Supportive relationships with adults
Stable personality
Having a special skill
High IQ and academic achievement
Parents who give high levels of supervision and clear discipline.

Assessment of psychiatric disorder in children

Evaluation of psychiatric disorder in very young children may seem to be inappropriate because thoughts and feelings are still developing and rapidly changing in this age group. Nevertheless, preschool children do experience strong emotions, which they communicate most expressively with their behaviour and their play. Thus, surveillance assessment of young children must focus most carefully on how the child behaves in various situations. An additional complicating factor in assessing younger children is that they tend to reflect the moods and attitudes of their main carer. The child–parent relationship and the mental state of the parent therefore form an important part of the assessment for psychiatric disorder.

Assessing children and their relationships is a complex process in which the observations of parents and teachers must play a major role. Information about the child must be gathered from as many sources as possible. Even so, a child's disturbance is often situation specific, with reports of problem behaviour in one setting only. Psychiatric disorders that are manifest in one situation only do not necessarily mean that the cause of the problem must also be there; a child may be difficult at home because of academic failure at school or may present major problems at school because of abuse at home.

The assessment process must therefore take account of the context in which the problems occur and note how each aetiological factor interacts with the others to generate the problem. It is helpful to start by considering the contribution that the child makes to the development of the disorder and then go on to review the role of the family and finally the influence of school and the outside world, as outlined in Boxes 1.2–1.5.

Screening for psychiatric disorder

Parents and teachers will always be a major source of information, but as children grow older it becomes increasingly relevant to obtain details from the children themselves. Most children younger than 7–8 years find it difficult to report their own feelings or to give a considered view of how they perceive the world. Nevertheless, it is always worthwhile directly questioning younger children to see what they have to say, provided that this is put in a developmental context. Accordingly, whatever the age of the child, it is important to use direct observation and questioning of the child, rather than to rely solely on the reports of others.

Questionnaires and rating scales can be used to screen children for psychiatric disorder. These are mostly aimed at parents and teachers, but new scales are now being developed for older children to rate their own symptoms. On the face of it, questionnaires might seem to be the answer to the problem of screening large numbers of children for psychiatric disorder, but caution is required because all scales are subject to error and throw up both false positive and false negative results. Young children can be assessed using the Preschool Behaviour Questionnaire.[1] School age children can be screened using the Strengths and Difficulties Questionnaire (SDQ), which is completed by parents, teachers and youngsters themselves; this scale measures common emotional and behavioural problems.[2] The SDQ is well established as a properly validated and reliable scale. It is short and easy to administer. A longer but equally well established schedule is the Child Behaviour Checklist.[3]

Early signs of psychiatric disorder

Adverse temperamental characteristics can be recognised soon after birth and are associated with an appreciable increase in the risk of behaviour problems developing at a later stage. Other factors, such as the appearance and sex of the child, will also play a role in determining parental perceptions and responses. The seeds for future parent–child relationship problems may be sown during this early stage, but it is important not to see these early experiences as fixed and unresponsive to outside influences.

The risk of poor early child care and parent–child relationship problems is increased if the mother has received poor child care herself. A parent who required special schooling for learning difficulties as a child, and very young parents are also likely to find child care a problem. Fortunately, deficiencies in mothering can be compensated for by a supportive father or other caring adult (Box 1.6).

Box 1.6 Factors that make child care more difficult

Unsupported single parent
Maternal depression
Limited parental intellectual ability (IQ less than 70%)
Teenage pregnancy
Poor parental relationship
Poor parenting experience as a child
Lack of parental involvement
Persistent rejection of the child after the first three months.

Although it is vital not to assume that there will inevitably be problems if one or more risk factors are present, careful surveillance should be maintained until it is clear that good progress is being made. Direct observation of parental behaviour with the baby is more reliable than what parents actually say. Surveillance during the first few weeks should therefore focus on parent–child interactions and should particularly note the parental responses listed in Box 1.7. Any problem that might be noted in the parent–child relationship at this early state is not necessarily serious – most parents will resolve any difficulties within a few months – but this early period is a critical time when support and encouragement for the more vulnerable parents can be especially effective.

Box 1.7 Checklist for assessing parenting of very young children

Feeding
Attending to basic child care tasks
Playing with and talking to the baby
Responding to distress and crying
Protecting from danger
Showing attention.

The preschool child

The range of emotional and behavioural symptoms is relatively limited in the preschool years. At this stage of rapid maturation any emotional or physical stress will cause obvious regression to more immature behaviour. It is therefore important not to be over-impressed by the apparently dramatic appearance of regressive behaviour during a physical illness, or with emotional distress or excitement. However, the behaviour should return to normal within a period of days or weeks once the stress is removed. A sound knowledge of child development is necessary to put any immaturity in perspective and thus distinguish between generally delayed development, specific developmental delay, and regression.

On starting primary school a child should have reached a reasonable level of social acceptability, and at this stage psychiatric disorders tend to present as immature behaviour. The main areas for psychiatric surveillance in preschool children are shown in Box 1.8.

Box 1.8 Checklist for preschool children

Feeding and sleeping patterns
Activity level and concentration
Bowel and bladder control
Temper and impulse control
Separation anxiety
Responsiveness to social cues
Ability to communicate basic needs.

Emotional and behavioural disorders in preschool children are relatively non-specific, and the range of normal behaviour is so great that it is often difficult to decide what is abnormal. It is best to adopt a pragmatic approach to diagnosing psychiatric disorder in preschool children, and it may help to pose the following simple question – is the child's reaction "out of proportion" to what might normally be expected in the circumstances, and is the child or the carer handicapped as a result?

The school age child

The role of parents and the family in generating psychiatric disorder is crucial in younger children, but as children grow older other factors gradually grow more important and the influence of the school and of other children becomes relatively greater. Surveillance at this stage needs to take into account what is happening at school and events outside the family in addition to the dynamics of the family itself.

Starting school is an important maturational experience. Children are assessed on their own merits in a more critical and detached way than most parents find possible. This may lead to temporary difficulties such as separation problems or disobedience. Appropriate management at school in liaison with the child's home should bring about a rapid resolution, thus distinguishing these transient difficulties from a more serious psychiatric disorder.

Young children are remarkably resilient, but as they grow older and become more self aware they are increasingly influenced by the attitudes of others. By age eight years most children have a reasonably clear view of themselves and how they compare with other youngsters. At this age a child can develop a sense of failure and a low self esteem, which will greatly increase the risk of emotional and behavioural problems.

Regression and immature behaviour are relatively more important if they occur in older children. For example, enuresis in children older than seven or eight years is likely to result in low self esteem, thereby making the child more vulnerable to failure in other areas of functioning, such as school work. Overactivity is another symptom that has added seriousness when it occurs in school age children. Inattentiveness and distractibility will interfere with learning, which in turn may provoke negative responses from teachers and other children. This can quickly result in a vicious cycle of failure, distress, opting out, and disruptive behaviour.

Surveillance for emotional and behavioural disorders in school age children should include those factors that are considered for younger children, but should also focus on more subtle areas of functioning, such as how the child manages relationships and the child's self perception and ability to control impulses. Academic achievement plays a critical role at this stage, and so the ability to concentrate and to read and write at an age appropriate level will strongly influence a child's mental state (Box 1.9).

Box 1.9 Checklist for school age children

Academic progress, especially ability to read
Relationships with adults and children
Self esteem
Concentration span
Mood state
Impulse control.

Symptoms that indicate serious psychopathology

Most psychiatric conditions in childhood are disorders of mental functioning and not illnesses. The distinction being that a disorder is an exaggeration of normal symptoms to the point that they become handicapping – a quantitative difference – whereas an illness is qualitatively different from normality. Thus, most emotional and behavioural symptoms are relatively non-specific, and the presence of a single symptom will give little intimation of the seriousness of the underlying psychopathology. It is the pattern of associated symptoms and the context in which they occur that give a better indication. However, some symptoms are strongly associated with definite psychiatric disorder, even when they occur in isolation. These symptoms are listed in Box 1.10 and should always be seen as having potentially serious implications, warranting detailed assessment and careful management.

Box 1.10 Checklist of potentially serious symptoms

Persistent deliberate destructiveness
Aggression leading to injury
Deliberate self harm
Sexual behaviour inappropriate to age
Fire setting
Social disinhibition
Persistent isolation and withdrawal
Bizarre behaviour
Hallucinations and delusions.

Symptoms with a particularly poor prognosis

The serious symptoms of mental dysfunction listed in Box 1.10 are indicative of pronounced psychopathology, but they do not necessarily mean a poor prognosis if appropriate treatment is provided at an early stage. There are, however, a few specific symptoms of childhood that have a particularly poor long term prognosis. These are listed in Box 1.11.

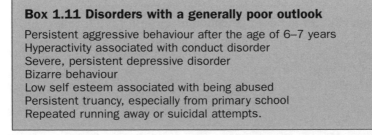

Box 1.11 Disorders with a generally poor outlook

Persistent aggressive behaviour after the age of 6–7 years
Hyperactivity associated with conduct disorder
Severe, persistent depressive disorder
Bizarre behaviour
Low self esteem associated with being abused
Persistent truancy, especially from primary school
Repeated running away or suicidal attempts.

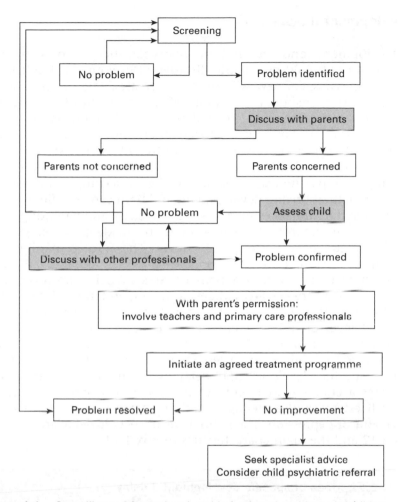

Figure 1.1   Surveillance of emotional and behavioural problems in children

After identification – what then?

A successful identification or surveillance programme will identify many children with psychiatric disorder. Awareness of their distress is only helpful if it leads to positive help and support. The issue of what to do with identified children needs to be agreed and planned well before any surveillance programme is started. A series of decisions must be made so that the most seriously disturbed children are provided with appropriate treatment. At the same time, it is necessary to avoid labelling children as being disturbed if the disorder is mild or likely to be transient. Figure 1.1 suggests the decision making steps and responses that can be taken as part of a surveillance process.

Developmental issues

Development and maturation play significant roles in the presentation of child psychiatric disorders. Development implies the addition of particular new skills or characteristics, whereas maturation indicates an increase or evolution of what is already there. For example, anger presents in an immature form in toddlers, in which there is little control or direction to a temper tantrum. Anger gradually matures with age, and becomes more controlled and better directed as the child grows older. On the other hand, skills such as walking and reading develop as new skills. Naturally, there is a complex interaction between maturation and development, and both can be influenced by environmental influences such as social adversity and parenting style.

There is an important distinction to be made between general developmental delay and specific delay. The former manifests as generalised learning difficulty (also known as mental handicap), with delays in every aspect of development. Specific delay, however, only affects one or a very few areas of development, and most of the child's development is satisfactory. This gap between the actual and the expected level of development needs to be at least 20%. Thus, a 10 year old child with specific delay in reading (dyslexia) would have a reading age of eight years or less in spite of at least average general ability. Specific developmental delay is an important factor that increases a child's vulnerability to mental health problems such as low self esteem and a feeling of failure that can lead to antisocial behaviour or depression. The main areas of specific delay are listed in Box 1.12 and the main characteristics in Box 1.13.

Box 1.12 Areas of specific developmental delay

Reading (dyslexia)
Motor control (dyspraxia)
Enuresis (and often encopresis)
Language and communication difficulties
Self control (attention deficit and hyperactivity disorder).

Box 1.13 Characteristics associated with specific developmental delay

More common in males – usually about 4 : 1
Tend to occur in families – probably both genetic and sociocultural influences
Follow a normal although slow developmental progress
Improve with time
Respond best to training approaches
Make the child especially vulnerable to stress
Become progressively more noticeable until the skill is acquired
Specific developmental delays tend to be associated with each other.

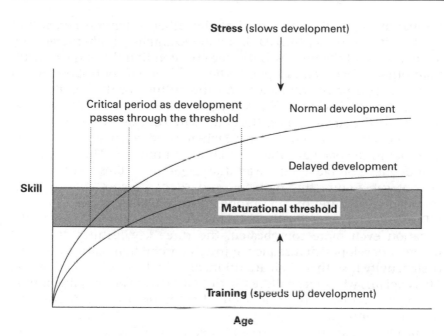

Figure 1.2 Skill development

The relationship between specific developmental delay and normal development is indicated in Figure 1.2. It is helpful to imagine a critical period during which a particular skill is being acquired. Once above the threshold, the skill has been achieved and any further development is in the form of maturation and consolidation. A skill is particularly vulnerable to physical and emotional stress when it is near the threshold. For example, a child who has just learnt to walk will easily "go off their legs" with any minor illness or upset. Training is especially important during the critical period; for example, a child who has not been introduced to solid food before the age of 3–4 years will have serious difficulty coping when it is introduced. The diagram also shows how the developmental gap increases with time.

At least 10% of children have a significant specific developmental delay but in Child and Adolescent Mental Health Services the rate may be more than 40%, indicating the increased vulnerability of these children. Figure 1.2 demonstrates how children with delayed development take longer to pass through the critical period during which problems with training are much more noticeable.

Continuum or spectrum disorders

There are a number of child psychiatric disorders that can be conceptualised as occurring along a developmental continuum from normal at one end to abnormal at the other. Attention deficit and hyperactivity disorder (ADHD) is a good example. Children gradually learn to control themselves, but some children find this more difficult than others. There comes a point where lack of self control becomes a problem. This point will depend on the attitude of the child's carers and anyone else directly affected by the child's behaviour. It will also depend on the circumstances the child is in. For example, there will be more problems in a confined space where good behaviour is expected than out in the open air where the child can run free. Thus, the point that defines a problem is quite arbitrary. Questionnaires and checklists do not get around this problem, and so it is important to get as rounded a picture of the problem as possible, using different informants and observing the child in different situations. To make the situation even more complicated, the three key features of ADHD follow a developmental sequence in which children learn to control their activity first, then their attention, and finally their impulsiveness. This explains why older children with ADHD may appear quite normal during a psychiatric assessment but show impulsiveness in everyday life. The only way to diagnose the condition is to note the characteristic pattern of symptoms in earlier childhood.

Another continuum disorder concerns problems with language development. The central problem is a specific difficulty in processing symbols that are used to communicate. This includes spelling, reading, spoken, and non-verbal language and "inner" language or thoughts. The most severe form of this difficulty is autism, followed by Asperger's syndrome, semantic pragmatic language disorder, and milder forms of receptive and expressive language difficulties. The boundary between each condition is fairly arbitrary and is often dealt with by lumping them together as "autistic spectrum disorder" (ASD). Unfortunately, this causes even more confusion because it covers such a wide range of disability from very mild to extreme handicap. Further problems can occur with different interpretations of severity, especially in the boundary area between normal and pathological. Consideration of the child's early developmental pattern can be helpful because there should be evidence of earlier communication difficulty. In view of the difficulty in deciding where to draw the line in order to diagnose a continuum disorder, it is not surprising that there are frequent misunderstandings and disputes when a diagnosis of ADHD or ASD is made. Because the disorders occur along a spectrum, it is all too easy to label children, who only have very mild symptoms, as suffering from the definitive condition.

Conclusion

The identification of mental health problems in children is a complex matter and must take a wide range of different factors into account. An overall rate for psychiatric disorder of 7–14% can be expected in the general child population. This means that many children will be identified in a surveillance process. However, not all of these children will require formal psychiatric assessment and treatment. Many can be helped by their parents and by appropriately skilled professionals. Informal psychiatric advice may be helpful at an early stage before a problem has become firmly established. Close collaboration with colleagues in the child psychiatry service is therefore important.

References

1   McGuire J, Richman N. Screening for behaviour problems in nurseries: the reliability and validity of the Preschool Behaviour Checklists. *J Child Psychol Psychiatry* 1986;**27**:7–32.
2   Goodman R. Strengths and Difficulties Questionnaire: a research note. *J Child Psychol Psychiatry* 1997;**38**:581–5.
3   Achenbach TM, Edelbrock C. *Manual for the Child Behaviour Checklist and revised child behavior profile*. Burlington, Vermont: University of Vermont, Department of Psychiatry, 1983.

Further reading

Goodman R, Scott S. *Child psychiatry*. Oxford: Blackwell Science, 2002. (An excellent short textbook)
Graham P, Turk J, Verhulst F, eds. *Child psychiatry: a developmental approach*. Oxford: Oxford University Press, 1999.

2: Types of psychiatric treatment

PHILIP GRAHAM

Overview

It is important that referrers to Child and Adolescent Mental Health Services (CAMHS) know what sort of management children and families are likely to receive.

Treatment involves managing the context of children's difficulties, in addition to individual treatment (psychological or physical), and group and family therapies.

CAMHS is the term currently most in favour to describe specialist child and adolescent psychiatric services, child and family centres or clinics, and child guidance clinics.

CAMHS teams are usually multidisciplinary and include child and adolescent psychiatrists, nurse therapists, clinical psychologists, social workers, and family and other therapists.

There is now a considerable evidence base for many of the treatments available for use in CAMHS.

Introduction

The aim of this chapter is to provide doctors and other practitioners, especially those practising in primary care and paediatrics, with an overview of therapeutic approaches used in departments of child and adolescent psychiatry. Such information is highly relevant because, among the children and adolescents seen in these settings, a large number have behavioural and emotional problems.[1,2] A small proportion will need referral to specialist services. It is important that referrers know what sort of management these children and their families are likely to receive. Many are not referred because the child psychiatric resources are inadequate, because parents are not motivated to attend specialist clinics, or because the disturbances, although bothersome, are not serious enough to merit referral. In these cases, the primary care doctor or paediatrician, or members of their teams may find it helpful to apply brief modifications to some of the forms of therapy described here (and, in more detail, in later chapters of this book), appropriately adapted to the settings in which they work. This may sound like encouragement of dangerous dabbling, but primary care doctors, paediatricians, and other practitioners need to be able to assess and provide help for families with disturbed children. Provided practitioners take opportunities for training, proceed with caution, are appropriately self critical, and have the opportunity to discuss what they are doing with a mental health professional from time to time, these modified approaches can be extremely helpful.

Definitions of treatment

Once they have assessed the nature of a problem, mental health professionals may try to alter the circumstances, or "context", in which behavioural difficulties occur. They can do this before specific therapies are undertaken or at the same time. "Managing the context" may take various forms, depending on what are thought to be the unique needs of the child (Box 2.1).

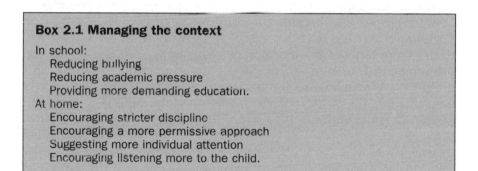

Box 2.1 Managing the context

In school:
  Reducing bullying
  Reducing academic pressure
  Providing more demanding education.
At home:
  Encouraging stricter discipline
  Encouraging a more permissive approach
  Suggesting more individual attention
  Encouraging listening more to the child.

The term *psychiatric treatment* covers all therapeutic approaches used in children with emotional and behavioural disturbances. Specific types of treatment can be divided into *psychological therapies* and *physical therapies* (Box 2.2). The indications and contraindications of the different types of treatment are discussed in other chapters of this book.

Box 2.2 Types of psychiatric treatment

Psychological:
  Behavioural
  Cognitive behavioural
  Psychodynamic, psychoanalytic.
Physical:
  Medication
  Diet.

Psychological therapies

Psychological therapies are termed *behavioural* if they aim to alter what the child or family do by methods that tackle the symptoms directly, without consideration of thoughts or feelings. For example, a specific phobia may be successfully treated by a desensitisation programme directed toward gradual familiarisation with the feared object in imagination or in real life.

Cognitive behavioural therapy aims to produce behavioural change by relating maladaptive patterns of thinking to behaviour, and *cognitive therapy* focuses exclusively on changing maladaptive thoughts. For example, depressive states may be maintained by false ideas about the way other people think about the patient. These may be influenced by encouraging the child to record the circumstances in which these thoughts occur and checking whether their beliefs are justified.

Psychological therapies also include those that aim to uncover underlying conflicts, tensions, and drives of which the child and family members were previously unaware and which are thought to be the covert source of the problem. For example, an anxiety state may have developed because the child has aggressive feelings toward a sibling that they have repressed and are unaware of until these feelings are uncovered by therapy. This may involve observing, listening, and talking or playing with the child. Such insight promoting therapies are termed *psychoanalytic* if they are clearly derived from the work of early psychoanalysts, especially Sigmund and Anna Freud and Melanie Klein. The term *psychoanalytic treatment* is usually reserved for quite intensive (3–5 times a week) individual treatment, and it is more likely to be termed *psychotherapy* or *psychodynamic therapy* if the underlying concepts are the same but treatment is provided on a less frequent basis. Much of once weekly or less frequent *counselling* uses a similar framework.

However, psychological therapies can also be classified according to the unit (individual, family, or group) to which therapy is applied. Those engaged in family therapy may use either psychodynamic or behavioural concepts, or a mixture of the two. They may also use concepts that are special to family therapists. Thus, *systems therapy* is based on the notion that families can be viewed as homeostatic entities – if you change one part of the system you alter the remainder.

Not so long ago there was considerable antagonism between psychodynamic therapists and behaviour therapists. Psychodynamic therapists saw behaviourism as superficial tinkering that left the real problems untouched. Behaviourists saw psychodynamic therapists as misguidedly applying an unproven set of theories, with little interest in or evidence for success. Such mutual dismissiveness has by no means disappeared, but there is distinctly more appreciation of the fact that different forms of treatment can be valuable in different circumstances.

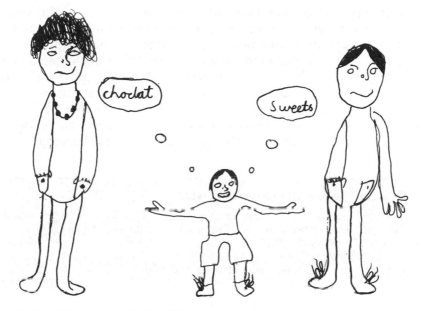

Psychiatric treatment can help children to develop more rewarding and trusting relationships with others

Physical therapies

Physical therapies are less commonly used in children. They include medication, dietary approaches, and electroconvulsive treatment, the latter of which is used either extremely rarely or not at all until late adolescence, and even then to a rapidly diminishing degree.

Other approaches

Child mental health professionals also provide indirect treatment through consultation without direct clinical contact. *Consultation and liaison work* is carried out especially with paediatricians, social workers, and teachers.

Finally, there are various miscellaneous forms of psychiatric treatment that cannot readily be classified according to the above system. *Hypnosis*, for example, aims to allow the child greater control of their behaviour by means of techniques used while they are in a state of altered awareness.

Treatment settings and staff

The structure of services for disturbed children and their families is illustrated in Box 2.3 (also see Chapter 11).[3] *Tier One* consists of primary care health professionals, especially family doctors and health visitors, as well as teachers and others who are in direct contact with children. *Tier Two* interventions are made especially by psychologists, nurses, or psychiatrists providing an individual service, either in a clinic or in the community. *Tier Three* services are more traditionally provided in child and family psychiatric clinics. *Tier Four* comprises specialist services such as those that target children with attention deficit and hyperactivity disorder (ADHD) or eating disorders. Inpatient services for children and adolescents are also included under this heading.

Box 2.3 The four tier model of services

Tier One: primary or direct contact services
Tier Two: interventions by individual staff of Child and Adolescent Mental
   Health Services (CAMHS)
Tier Three: interventions by CAMHS teams
Tier Four: very specialised interventions and care.

Tier Three services used to be termed Child Guidance Clinics if they were sited in the community or Child and Adolescent Psychiatry Clinics if based in hospitals. It is now much more common for them to be variously termed, for example, Child and Adolescent Centre or Child and Family Consultation Service. Child and Adolescent Mental Health Services (CAMHS) is increasingly becoming the generic term.

Child and adolescent departments of psychiatry or mental health may be sited in general hospitals, psychiatric hospitals, children's hospitals, or in the community. Inpatient units usually admit either children who are from 6–7 years old up to early adolescence, or they admit older adolescents. Some units for young adults will also admit older adolescents. Inpatient units may admit a proportion of day patients, and there is a relatively small number of child psychiatric day centres exclusively given over to day patients. Many CAMHS staff work in other settings, such as schools for children with emotional and behaviour disorders (EBD schools) and child development clinics, or with social services.

Professional teams working in any of these centres are likely to be multidisciplinary, and treatment may be delivered by any of the professionals involved. Child and adolescent psychiatrists have particular skills in formulating clinical problems in which both biological and psychosocial factors are important. Among CAMHS staff, they alone will be able to prescribe psychotropic medication. They are usually the gatekeepers for inpatient treatment.

As well as child and adolescent psychiatrists, who are medically trained, the team is likely to include clinical psychologists. Although traditionally psychologists have spent much time systematically testing children, they now spend a much greater proportion of their time assessing children and families, and then devising and sometimes carrying out programmes of treatment. Educational psychologists (who have all had teaching experience) do not usually form part of the CAMHS team but rather work in the educational service, often spending much time processing statements of special educational need. Especially in London and the Home Counties, although increasingly elsewhere too, family therapists and other creative therapists work as part of the CAMHS team. Although many local authority social workers remain in child and family psychiatric clinics and departments, some have been withdrawn and others are mainly occupied with child protection and court work, and have little or no time for therapy. Some, however, have retrained as family therapists.

Child psychiatrists and clinical psychologists are likely to apply a range of therapeutic techniques, including most of those described above. In addition, an important and relatively new development is the presence of child psychiatric nurses. Although they still most frequently work in inpatient units or day centres, these are now increasingly likely to exercise their skills in the community. Family therapists have special training in therapies that include all family members. Although child psychotherapists have a very specialised training in individual psychoanalytic techniques, they are increasingly involved in liaison work and sometimes family work. They may be attached to primary care clinics or paediatric outpatient clinics.

Is child psychiatric treatment effective?

There is increasing emphasis throughout medical practice on the need to provide treatment that is evidence based. The degree to which one can state that child psychiatric treatment is based on good evidence depends on the definition of evidence, on the particular diagnosis, and on the nature of the intervention.[4] Before describing specific forms of therapy, it is worth remembering that all therapy will be more effective if the practitioner shows the characteristics of genuineness, trust, and empathy, which were shown 50 years ago to be essential for therapeutic success.[5] Such features of the therapist go far to explain the success of alternative forms of therapy that are not described here because the empirical evidence for their effectiveness is lacking.

Medication

It is relatively easy to conduct double blind, randomised controlled studies with medication. There is strong evidence from rigorously conducted trials for the effectiveness of stimulant medication in children with ADHD or hyperkinetic disorder.[6] A minority of children with ADHD respond to dietary interventions.[7] There is a small number of trials with positive results using selective serotonin reuptake inhibitors in adolescent depression.[8] However, most justification for the use of this medication comes from trials conducted in adults. In contrast, it seems that tricyclic antidepressants are ineffective in reducing depression in this age group, although they may reduce anxiety and act as hypnotics. The severe tics that occur in Tourette syndrome are reduced with neuroleptic medication, although side effects often limit its value.

Cognitive and cognitive behavioural therapies

Psychological therapies are much more difficult to evaluate using controlled designs, but recently considerable progress has been made in this direction.[9] A number of studies have been conducted in children, and this approach has been demonstrated to be effective in a variety of conditions. Thus, some young children with conduct disorders, especially if these are of mild or moderate severity, respond to parent management training.[10] Severe conduct disorders are improved with so-called multisystem therapy. Cognitive behaviour therapy is an effective treatment for some depressive and anxiety disorders, as well as for obsessive–compulsive states and post-traumatic stress disorder. Monosymptomatic phobias respond to behavioural treatment, and the bell and pad alarm is another form of behaviour therapy that is effective in nocturnal enuresis.

Psychoanalytic psychotherapy and counselling

It is difficult to distinguish between these two approaches, but in general counselling is likely to involve a higher component of advice and guidance, with less dependence on a theoretical model involving the presence of unconscious mechanisms. Psychoanalytic psychotherapy is probably effective in some diffuse anxiety states.[11] Family therapy has been shown to be effective in a variety of conditions.[12] It appears, for example, to reduce the frequency of attacks in childhood asthma and, when combined with other approaches, to be an effective intervention in anorexia nervosa.

Factors that impact on the effectiveness of treatment

For some common disorders, it remains likely that non-specific factors such as the enthusiasm of the therapist and the motivation of family members are of greater importance than the specific type of treatment employed. Paediatricians and general practitioners in training who find themselves working with psychiatrists and psychologists with different therapeutic orientations may be confused, but should find that they can learn much that is of value from observing the application of different approaches to similar problems. In particular, they may benefit as much from observing how child mental health professionals can clarify the nature of a problem, helping the child and family to see their difficulties in a new way, as they can from observing specific treatment interventions.

As the classification systems used in child psychiatry become more refined, there will probably be increased precision in our application of different forms of treatment. In the meantime, it would be highly desirable for evaluative studies to include not only scientifically valid controlled trials but also measures of consumer satisfaction. With increasing dependence on their "customers", among whom they must certainly count those working in primary care and paediatric settings, child mental health professionals will be increasingly sensitive to what their clients think of their interventions.

Which children should be referred?

The indications for referral to a child and adolescent psychiatric service are listed in Box 2.4.

> **Box 2.4 Indications for referral to a child and adolescent psychiatric service**
>
> Children with active suicidal thoughts or psychotic symptoms
> Emotional or behaviour problems not responding to first line counselling
> Difficult diagnostic problems with no obvious organic cause.

Where there is provision of a Tier Two consultation service (see Box 2.3), with specialist staff coming out to advise and sometimes see children and families in the paediatric outpatient clinic or the community based primary health care centre, referral to a child mental health service is not really a problematic issue.[13] There will always be the opportunity for discussion of potential referrals. For those with less close contacts, some guidance may be helpful.

Children with moderately severe behaviour or emotional problems or with disabling psychosomatic symptoms should be referred to a child mental health service if the problems do not resolve after first line counselling. Children who are appreciably functionally disabled by persistent physical problems that either have no organic basis or an insufficient organic explanation need referral, and the earlier they are referred the better. Similarly, children with active suicidal thoughts or psychotic symptoms should be referred urgently. When, in a paediatric clinic, it is clear from the time of first attendance that children presenting with difficult diagnostic problems probably have a non-organic explanation for their symptoms, then again the children should be referred early on – preferably while physical investigations are still being carried out. This is so that when all results prove negative (as is highly likely to happen in these circumstances), the child psychiatric department is not seen as a last resort or "dustbin" department. Instead, the child psychiatrist is seen as someone who has been involved from the start. In the very occasional child who turns out to have an abdominal tumour or a degenerative neurological condition to explain, for example, severe stomach aches or headaches, the early involvement of a psychiatrist need not antagonise parents if it is made clear at the outset that the diagnostic process may indeed show an organic cause.

Of course, only a minority of primary health care physicians and paediatricians are able to refer to a CAMHS as much as they would wish. Those who press energetically for an increase in their child psychiatric and psychological services will usually obtain better resources within a reasonable period of time. The gradual emergence of stronger clinical child psychology and community child psychiatric nursing services is allowing child and adolescent psychiatrists to concentrate more on the hospital and community work for which their medical and psychiatric training has specifically equipped them.

References

1 Kramer T, Garralda E. Psychiatric disorders in adolescents in primary care. *Br J Psychiatry* 1998;**173**:508–13.
2 Appleton P, Hammond-Rowley S. Addressing the population of child and adolescent mental health problems: a primary care model. *Child Psychol Psychiatry Rev* 2000;**5**:9–16.
3 Health Advisory Service. *Together we stand: the commissioning, role and management of Child and Adolescent Mental Health Services*. London: HMSO, 1995.
4 Graham P. Treatment interventions and findings from research: bridging the chasm in child psychiatry. *Br J Psychiatry* 2000;**176**:414–9.
5 Rogers C. *Client centred therapy in current practice: implications and theory*. New York: Houghton Mifflin, 1951.
6 Taylor E, Sergeant J, Doepfner M, *et al*. Clinical guidelines for hyperkinetic disorder. *Eur Child Adolesc Psychiatry* 1998;**7**:184–200.
7 Carter C, Urbanowicz M, Hemsley R, *et al*. Effects of a few foods diet in attention deficit disorder. *Arch Dis Child* 1993;**69**:564–8.
8 Emslie GJ, Rush AJ, Weiberg WA, *et al*. A double blind, randomised placebo-controlled trial of fluoxetine in children and adolescents with depression. *Arch Gen Psychiatry* 1997;**54**:1031–7.
9 Graham P, ed. *Cognitive behaviour therapy for children and families*. Cambridge: Cambridge University Press, 1998.
10 Webster-Stratton C, Hammond M. Treating children with early onset conduct problems: a comparison of child and parent training interventions. *J Consult Clin Psychol* 1997;**65**:93–109.
11 Fonagy P, Target M. Predictors of outcome in child psychoanalysis: a retrospective study of 763 cases at the Anna Freud Centre. *J Am Psychoanal Assoc* 1996;**44**:27–77.

12 Shadish W, Montgomery L, Wilson P, Wilson M, Bright I, Okumabua T. The effects of family and marital psychotherapies: a meta-analysis. *J Consult Clin Psychol* 1993;**61**:992–1002.

13 Subotsky F, Brown R. Working alongside the general practitioner: a child psychiatric clinic in the general practice setting. *Child Care Health Dev* 1997;**16**:189–96.

Further reading

Goodman R, Scott S. *Child psychiatry*. Oxford: Blackwell, 1997.

Graham P, Turk J, Verhulst F. *Child psychiatry: a developmental approach*, 3rd edn. Oxford: Oxford University Press, 1999.

Section II
Treatments

3: Parenting programmes

STEPHEN SCOTT

Overview

Parents do not necessarily know "naturally" how to handle children, but can learn well.

Causes of difficulty may include child factors such as temperament and hyperactivity, rather than just parental considerations.

Outcomes for children brought up by critical, harsh parents are quite poor in terms of their ability to succeed and gain satisfaction from either work or relationships.

Scores of controlled trials have shown that behaviourally based parenting programmes are effective in reducing poor parenting practices and increasing child social behaviour.

Successful programmes stress the promotion of a positive relationship with the child, rather than only teaching more effective discipline; once a positive relationship is in place, many behavioural difficulties disappear anyway.

Evaluations of humanistic, counselling type parenting programmes show that, although they are often well received by parents, they are frequently ineffective in changing parenting practices or improving child behaviour.

There is a need for further training of professionals and voluntary organisations in programmes that are effective, and for inculcation of a culture of evaluation of outcomes.

Self administered programmes using books and videotapes can be surprisingly effective for suitably motivated parents.

Introduction

This chapter addresses proven, systematic approaches to helping parents who are having difficulty managing their children's behaviour. This can have important consequences because such parents often end up exhausted, and can become depressed. Their child's behaviour in public can make them feel shamed, and at home it can put a strain on their marriage, and over time it may make them increasingly punitive toward their child as they try to assert control. In some cases children whose behaviour has been highly frustrating to parents may become the target of parental bitterness and hatred, and be blamed for ruining their parents' lives.

There is now good evidence that such inappropriate parenting practices have a permanent effect on child outcome. Children exposed

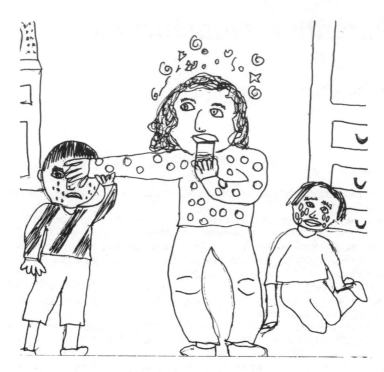

Harsh and neglectful parenting can be linked with delinquency in the child

to high levels of criticism and hostility grow up to be far less confident and do less well. One UK study[1] found that individuals who had highly critical or hostile mothers at age 10 grew up to have much poorer self esteem as adults. This affected their enjoyment of life, the kind of partners they ended up with, and how successful they were at their jobs. Many child disorders are worsened by negative parenting, and there is strong evidence to suggest that oppositional defiant disorder and other forms of antisocial behaviour are actively *caused* by inappropriate parenting.[2] Conduct disorder is the psychiatric label[3] for children who are persistently antisocial; for example, they fight excessively, are destructive, constantly disobedient, and may lie or steal.[4] Such children do poorly in terms of adult outcomes, with high rates of criminality, violent interpersonal relationships, and poor academic and work achievements.

In cases in which the parenting is frankly abusive, there is the risk of physical sequelae such as fractures and failure to thrive because physical and emotional abuse frequently coexist. For any professional, the question then arises at what point they are bound under the

Children Act (1989) to alert social services to investigate the family. For less severe parenting difficulties, the professional needs to know what can be done, and where the parents can find help.

How parents can cause behaviour problems in children

Fine grained analysis by Patterson[5] has shown that the moment to moment responses of parents toward children have a powerful effect on their behaviour. In families with difficulties, the children are often ignored when they are behaving reasonably but criticised and shouted at when they are misbehaving. The consequence is that, in order to gain attention, they must behave badly. What is perhaps surprising is that they prefer negative attention to none at all, and are prepared to elicit often unpleasant and frankly painful reactions from their parents. By contrast, children who receive a reasonable amount of positive attention within the family tend not to behave in a way that elicits negative attention. All of this can be summarised as the "attention rule", which states that children will behave in whatever way necessary to gain a reasonable amount of attention.

Other behaviours by parents can unwittingly raise the probability of disruptive behaviour in the child. Giving up insisting that something unpleasant is carried out (for example, tidying up the toys) unintentionally rewards the child for whining and refusing to do it, thus making whining and refusing more likely the next time a request is made. Giving in to demands for something pleasant (for example, sweets) has the same effects.

To date most emphasis in social learning theory has been on the harmful effect of negative behaviour. However, more recently research[6] has made it clear that the presence of positive parental behaviour is equally important. Children with antisocial behaviour are ignored for much of the time by their parents, who do not respond to their overtures to join in activities or praise them when they are behaving well. Not only does this make quiet activity less likely because no attention is forthcoming, but also no models are provided from which the child may learn social skills such as turn taking and negotiating skills.

The implications of the power of the interaction patterns are far-reaching. Rather than construing the child as innately aggressive or with an antisocial type of personality that is unchangeable, the child can be seen as responding to the immediate context that he or she is in. Change the context, and you will change the behaviour of the child. This can occur over minutes or hours. It allows some therapeutic optimism, because if the response contingencies around the child are altered then improvement can occur.

Applications of parenting programmes

Behaviourally based parenting programmes have repeatedly been shown in well conducted trials to be effective in improving parenting practices and child behaviour. The content of a typical modern programme is described below (summarised in Box 3.1); more detailed descriptions are available.[7,8]

Box 3.1 Key elements of a parenting programme

Promoting appropriate child behaviours through:
  Play
  Praise and rewards.
Reducing inappropriate behaviours through:
  Clear instructions
  Consequences of disobedience
  Ignore and distract
  Time out (from positive reinforcement).
Preventing difficulties arising through:
  Recognising patterns and planning ahead
  Listening and compromising
  Helping the child to become a problem solver
  Managing situations that occur
  General dimensions of parenting.

First part of a parenting programme: promoting appropriate child behaviour

Play

Most programmes start with play, which is perhaps the most fundamental aspect of improving the relationship with the child. Parents are asked to follow the child's lead rather than impose their own ideas. Instead of giving directions, teaching, and asking questions during play, parents are instructed simply to describe what the child is doing, to give a running commentary on their child's actions. The target is to give at least four of these "descriptive comments" per minute. If the parent has difficulty in getting going, the practitioner suggests precisely what they should do, for example by saying, "I'd like you to say to Adam 'You've picked up the yellow brick'". As soon as the parent has done this, the practitioner gives feedback – "That was a good descriptive comment".

After 10–15 minutes, this directly supervised play ends and the parent is "debriefed" for half an hour or more alone with the clinician. How the parent felt while doing it is explored, and reservations and difficulties that arose are addressed. Usually, the effect of their behaviour on the child during the training session is soon observed by the parent. Typically, the child is seen to settle and spend longer than usual playing purposefully with one game, rather than rushing round the room switching inconsequentially from one activity to another. Misbehaviour is usually at a lower level than normal. Experiencing this close, non-judgemental attention is surprisingly powerful for children, who at best feel they are "the apple of their parent's eye". For parents who have got to a state of affairs in which virtually all communication with the child is nagging and complaining, play is an important first step in mending the relationship. It often helps the parent to realise that it can be fun to be together with their child, and to begin to have positive feelings for the child again. Parents are asked to do homework by playing with their child using these techniques for 10 minutes every day.

At the second session a week later, the previous week's "homework" of playing at home is gone over with the parent in considerable detail for 20 minutes. Often there are practical reasons for not doing it ("I have to look after the other children, I've got no help"), and parents are then encouraged to solve the problem and find ways around the difficulty. (Solutions arrived at might include doing the play after the younger sibling has gone to bed; getting the oldest child to look after the baby while the parent plays with the toddler; and asking the parent's sister to come in to cover for the 15 minute play time.) With other parents there may be emotional blocks ("It feels wrong – no one ever played with me as a child") that need to be overcome before the parent feels able to practise the homework. By going over whatever the difficulty may be and gently pushing for a solution to try out, parents see that the clinician is quietly determined to have the changes implemented. In a way, the parents themselves are testing out the practitioner to see what will happen if they (rather than their child) do not comply with the rules. Getting over the hump of inertia is often very energising – the parents feel better for getting something done.

After this, the live session with the child is carried out. Usually, this continues where the previous one left off, and further develops the parent's play skills. This time the parent is encouraged to go beyond describing the child's behaviour and to make comments describing the child's likely mood state; for example, "You're really trying hard making that tower" or "That puzzle is making you really fed up". This process has benefits for both the parent and the child. The parent gets better at observing the fine details of the child's behaviour and this makes them more sensitive to the child's mood. This ability is important if responsive parenting is to develop, and it is poorly developed in unskilled parents[9]; thus, the problem is a perceptual one as well as a lack of skills. The child feels appreciated for what they are doing, and knows that their efforts and disappointments are appreciated. Through this process the child gradually gets better at understanding and labelling their own emotional states, which is a crucial step in gaining self control in frustrating situations. A feature of out of control children brought up in insensitive parenting environments is their inability to describe their emotions, often at the most basic level (so-called "alexithymia").

All subsequent sessions follow the same pattern of:

- reviewing the previous week's homework
- direct training of interaction with the child
- discussion afterward of how it went.

The speed at which the content is covered depends on progress.

Praise and rewards

A motto for this part of the programme is "catch them being good" and then praise them. Empirical studies show that, in families in which parents are having difficulty controlling their children, when the child does behave sociably he or she is ignored.[5] As a consequence, the only way for the child to gain attention is through being naughty. This leads to a situation in which the parent is unwittingly actively training their child to be antisocial. Reversal of this state of affairs requires the parents to praise their child for lots of mundane, everyday behaviours such as playing quietly on their own, eating nicely, getting dressed the first time they are asked, and so on. In this way the frequency of desired behaviour increases. However, many parents find this difficult. First, they may say, "But he *should* be doing these things anyway, without being praised for it – there's really no need". Second, when their child has misbehaved earlier in the day they are still cross, and this prevents them praising good behaviour when it occurs. Third, some parents find that even when they want to praise their child the whole process feels alien to them. Often they never experienced praise themselves as a child. In this situation a direct one to one intervention is invaluable, because the clinician can rehearse with the parent precisely how to speak to the child. Usually, with practice it becomes easier.

Second part of a parenting programme: reducing inappropriate behaviour

Clear instructions

A hallmark of ineffective parenting is a continuing stream of ineffectual, nagging demands for the child to do something. In the programme, parents are taught to reduce the number of such demands but to make them much more authoritative. This is done through altering both the manner in which they are given and what is said. The manner should be forceful (not sitting down, timidly requesting from the other end of the room; instead, standing over the child, fixing them in the eye, and in a clear firm voice giving the instruction). The emotional tone should be calm, without shouting or criticism. The content should be phrased directly ("I want you to …") and not indirectly or as a question ("Wouldn't you like to …"). It should be specific, labelling the desired behaviour in a way that the child can understand, so that it is clear to the child when he or she has complied ("Keep the sand in the box", rather than a vague "Do be tidy"). It should be simple (one action at a time, not a chain of orders) and performable immediately. Commands should be phrased as what the parent *does* want the child to do, not as what the child should *stop* doing ("Please speak quietly", rather than "Stop shouting"). If a child is in the middle of an activity, rather than abruptly ordering a stop, a warning should be given ("In two minutes you'll have to go to bed"). Rather than threatening the child with vague, dire consequences ("You're going to be sorry you did that"), *when–then* commands should be given ("When you've laid the table, then you can watch TV").

Consequences for disobedience

Consequences for disobedience should be applied as soon as possible. They must always be followed through; children quickly learn to calculate the probability that they will be applied, and if in fact a sanction is only given every third occasion then a child is being taught that he or she can misbehave the rest of the time. Simple logical consequences should be devised and enforced for everyday situations – if water is splashed out of the bath then the bath will end; if a child refuses to eat dinner then there will be no pudding. The consequences should "fit the crime", should not be punitive, and should not be long term (no bike riding for a month) because this will lead to a sense of hopelessness in the child who may see no point in behaving well if it seems there is nothing to gain. Planning ahead and giving the child a warning enables them to have an element of choice in their behaviour, and teaches them that they have a measure of control over the situation ("If you haven't picked up the toys by seven o'clock, there'll be no snack or story"). Consistency of enforcement is central.

Ignore and distract

This sounds easy but it is a hard skill to teach parents. Whining, arguing, swearing, and tantrums are not dangerous to children and other people and can usually safely be ignored. The technique is very effective when applied. Children soon realise that they are getting no payoff for the behaviours and soon stop. Vice versa, if acting in this way gets them attention and shows them that they can annoy and wind up their parents, then they will continue to hone their skills in so doing. Ignoring means avoiding discussion, avoiding eye contact, and turning away, but staying in the room to monitor. As soon as the child begins to behave appropriately, it is essential to attend and give praise. This is central to shaping up desirable behaviour – ignoring will only reduce undesirable behaviour, which is not the same thing. Many parents find this difficult because they are often still angry with the child. Distraction is useful with 2–4 year olds; after ignoring for some moments, an interesting alternative activity that is likely to capture the child's imagination is offered.

Time out

The full name of this is "time out from positive reinforcement". The point is to put the child in some boring place away from a reasonably pleasant context. This will not be the case if the home is generally negative, when being sent to a room alone will be a relief and not a punishment. Equally, if the room has lots of interesting toys then the same will apply. Time out should be in a boring place (such as the end of the corridor, porch, or toilet) for a previously agreed reason (for example, hitting or breaking things, not minor infringements) and for a short period (for example, a minute for each year of age). However, the child must be quiet for the last minute; if the child is still screaming, then they stay in the boring place for as long as it takes until they have been quiet for a minute. For the first few times, this may be for 30–40 minutes or more as the child tests out the new system. However, soon the period will reduce to a few minutes only. Parents must resist responding to taunts and cries from the child during time out because this will reinforce the child by giving attention. Time out provides a break for the adult to calm down also. At the end of the period, the child has received his or her punishment and should not be scolded. If the reason for the time out was failure to carry out an instruction, then the instruction should be given again (otherwise the child is being taught that, by disobeying, he can avoid complying). Time out should not need to be used more than a few times a week. If the child is spending more than about two hours per week in time out, then something is going wrong and the situation needs investigating. Most children are sent there for only a few minutes a week or not at all – the knowledge that it is there is often enough to help the child to comply.

Third part of a parenting programme: preventing difficulties arising

Recognising patterns and planning ahead

Parents are taught to keep a diary of when problem behaviours occur, what led up to them, and what happened afterward (the "ABC" of behaviour: antecedents, behaviour, consequences). They learn from this that tantrums do not occur randomly (although they used to appear that way), but that there are certain high risk situations and times. They learn to recognise their own role after the event in reinforcing the bad behaviour. By rearranging the child's schedule, many difficult situations can be avoided. A grandmother can look after the child during supermarket trips, a shower may be substituted for a bath, and long phone calls to friends may be made in the evening, and so on.

Listening and compromising

It is surprising how many parents are ignorant of their child's fears and main desires, as well as expectations in everyday situations. Children are seen as difficult because they will not do as they are told. However, often in fact they are subject to a bewildering flow of unreasonable demands and are frustratingly cut short without warning when they are quietly enjoying an activity. Getting parents to stop and listen to their child's wishes and fears is often a revelation for them. Then, negotiating how to accommodate the child's wishes while fitting in with the family goals for the day is practised. Having been consulted about the plan and contributed to it usually leads the child to behave more calmly and contentedly.

Helping the child to become a problem solver

This is another strategy that helps to stop impulsive reactions to frustration in children and helps them to slow down and devise their own solutions. Over the longer term this promotes independence. There are programmes of this kind taught directly by professionals to children,[10] but one can also get parents to use the process with their children. This has the advantage of getting the parents to think this way too. *Step 1* involves stopping to hear the child's side of the story. For *step 2*, the child is encouraged to generate as many solutions as possible to the problem, however silly (hit him/take his toy/run away), leading to some more sensible ones (offer him another toy instead). In *step 3*, each solution is evaluated for its pros and cons (if you hit him, he'll cry and not want you back in his house again). In *step 4*, the best option is chosen and carried out. Finally, for *step 5*, the solution is reviewed for its effectiveness and amended as necessary.

Managing situations that recur

There are several recurring situations in which a child's behaviour may be especially difficult for a family (for example, mealtimes, out in public, when the parent is on the telephone, difficulties going to bed and waking at night, lying and stealing, and sibling rivalry). Managing these can be practised in advance with a range of the strategies described above.

General dimensions of parenting

Several more strategic aspects beyond moment to moment interaction are covered. These include supervision and how this changes with age (for example, for how long should a three year old be out of view – no more than two minutes?; how does the parent set up their activities to enable this level of monitoring?; should an eight year old be allowed to play with another child for half an hour on the way home from school?), planning joint activities, reducing sibling rivalry, promoting friendships with other children, and how to deal with school and teachers.

Individual or group work?

Individual work

For severe difficulties, an individualised approach in which the parent and child are seen together allows one to go at the pace of the parent, observe precisely how they are relating to their child, and modify the intervention accordingly. This can be especially helpful where the child responds differently from the majority (for example, if the child is hyperactive, has a hearing or learning disability, or has autistic traits). An individualised approach also enables one to do more work on other issues that impinge on parenting, such as interparental consistency, sibling relationships, and coming to terms with abuse in the parent's own childhood. There is plentiful evidence from controlled trials of effectiveness.[11]

Group work

For moderately severe difficulties a group approach working with parents alone can be effective. The programme used in our clinic comprises a two-hour session once a week over 12 weeks for parents of six to eight children. Videotapes are shown of parents handling their children in the "right" and "wrong" ways, and then parents are invited to role play these in the group and practise them at home.[7] The advantages of the group approach are cost effectiveness and the support parents give each other. The disadvantages are that parents are not seen directly with their children, and there is little opportunity to explore deeper personal issues for the parent in front of the group. A recently completed controlled trial in the UK showed large effects in improving the problems parents were concerned with, as well as much reduced child antisocial behaviour.[12] The programme worked well with multiply disadvantaged families with severely antisocial children.

Self administered programmes

Because parenting programmes may be hard to access, the availability of do-it-yourself programmes is a boon. Most of the well known programmes have self administered versions with handouts or a book for parents.[13,14] Evaluations have shown they can be effective. In the UK, sending parents a book and then offering regular telephone advice led to reasonable gains on parent questionnaires and direct observation in two studies conducted by Sutton.[15,16] In a larger study conducted in the USA by Webster-Stratton,[17] parents were invited to come into the clinic regularly and follow the self administered version of her videotape series, with clinicians on hand to offer help if requested. Good gains were found on parent report compared with waiting list control. However, further research is needed to determine whether more disadvantaged families can benefit, perhaps with the addition of telephone calls. This mode of delivery has the potential to be a cost effective way to disseminate parenting programmes to a much wider section of the population.

Contraindications

There are no absolute contraindications, but caution should be exercised before immediately embarking on parenting work. Above all, a reasonable assessment of the child and family should be undertaken so that coexisting conditions that require other treatments are not missed. These include severe hyperactivity warranting consideration of medication, generalised learning disability, autistic traits, and speech and language problems. Disruptive behaviour can be the presenting complaint for all of these conditions. Parenting programmes could well be beneficial but should be used in addition to appropriate treatment for the coexisting condition.

Evidence base

There have been hundreds of trials of parenting programmes for disruptive behaviour, and several readable reviews.[11,18–22] From these it can be concluded that behaviourally based programmes are very effective, with a large effect size even in everyday practice with severe cases.[12] However, some caution is necessary because not all programmes are the same, nor are they all delivered with the same degree of skill or fidelity to the original plan. General parent counselling and support produces little change in child antisocial behaviour, even though parents may be satisfied with the experience.[23,24] The most effective programmes do address parental feelings and beliefs and use a collaborative approach,[25] but they also offer parents a whole range of specific strategies to deal with their children. Likewise, where the quality of implementation falls, so does the effectiveness.[26] Not only do programmes improve child behaviour and hyperactivity, but they also improve parenting quality and maternal depression, where present.

Potential for multi-agency application

Currently, there are insufficient places on evidence-based parenting programmes to meet demand. However, their availability is increasing fairly rapidly, and at the time of writing the National Institute for Clinical Excellence (NICE) is due to report on whether such programmes should be part of regular health care provision. Even if NICE does recommend them, the National Health Service will still have inadequate funds to meet the demand. Fortunately, several other agencies and projects are becoming involved. Thus, in deprived areas, the SureStart initiative is providing parenting programmes, and across the UK several voluntary organisations are doing so too.[27] They can best be accessed through the Parenting Education and Support Forum – the umbrella body for voluntary sector parenting programmes providers.[28]

Conclusion

Rigorous evaluation using randomised controlled trials has shown that behaviourally based parenting programmes considerably improve both the quality of parenting experienced and the behaviour and outcome for the child. Effective programmes address both the moment to moment minutiae of parents' handling of children and the wider context of their lives, which can get in the way of good enough parenting. The task now is to disseminate effective interventions and convince purchasers of their cost effectiveness and human value.

References

1 Maughan B, Pickles A, Quinton D. Parental hostility, childhood behavior, and adult social functioning. In: McCord J, ed. *Coercion and punishment in long-term perspectives*. Cambridge: Cambridge University Press, 1995.

2 Rutter M, Giller H, Hagell A. *Antisocial behavior by young people*. New York: Cambridge University Press, 1998.

3 WHO. *The ICD-10 Classification of Mental and Behavioural Disorders: clinical descriptions and diagnostic guidelines*. Geneva: World Health Organization, 1992.

4 Goodman R, Scott S. *Child psychiatry*. Oxford: Blackwell, 1997.

5 Patterson GR. *Coercive family process*. Eugene, OR: Castalia, 1982.

6 Gardner FME. Positive interaction between mothers and conduct-problem children: is there training for harmony as well as fighting? *J Abnorm Child Psychol* 1987;15:283–93.

7 Webster-Stratton C, Hancock L. Training for parents of young children with conduct problems: content, methods, and therapeutic processes. In: Briesmeister JM, Schaefer CE, eds. *Handbook of parent training*, 2nd edn. New York, NY: Wiley, 1998.

8 Barkley R. *Defiant children: a clinician's manual for assessment and parent training*, 2nd edn. New York, NY: Guilford, 1997.

9 Wahler RG, Dumas JE. Attentional problems in dysfunctional mother–child interactions: an interbehavioral model. *Psychol Bull* 1989;105:116–30.

10 Blomquist ML, Schnell SV. *Helping children with aggression and conduct problems*. London: Guilford, 2002.

11 Kazdin A. Psychosocial treatments for conduct disorder in children. *J Child Psychol Psychiatry* 1997;38:161–78.

12 Scott S, Spender Q, Doolan M, Jacobs B, Aspland H. Multicentre controlled trial of parenting groups for child antisocial behaviour in clinical practice. *BMJ* 2001;323:194–7.

13 Forehand RL, Long N. *Parenting the strong-willed child: the clinically proven five-week program for parents of two- to six-year-olds*. Chicago, IL: Contemporary Books, 1996.

14 Webster-Stratton C. *The incredible years: a trouble-shooting guide for parents of children aged 3–8*. Toronto, ON: Umbrella Press, 1992.

15 Sutton C. Training parents to manage difficult children: a comparison of methods. *Behav Psychother* 1992;20:115–39.

16 Sutton C. Parent training by telephone: a partial replication! *Behav Cogn Psychother* 1995;23:1–24.

17 Webster-Stratton C. Randomized trial of two parent-training programs for families with conduct-disordered children. *J Consult Clin Psychol* 1984;52:666–78.

18 Scott S. Parent training programmes. In: Rutter M, Taylor E, eds. *Child and adolescent psychiatry*, 4th edn. Oxford: Blackwell Science, 2002.

19 Fonagy P, Target M, Cottrell D, Phillips J, Kurtz Z. *What works for whom: a critical review of treatments for children and adolescents*. New York, NY: Guilford Press, 2002.

20 Carr A. *What works for children and adolescents?* London: Routledge, 2000.

21 Richardson J, Joughin C. *Parent training programmes for the management of young children with conduct disorders*. London: Gaskell, 2002.

22 Barlow J. *Systematic review of the effectiveness of parent-training programmes in improving behaviour problems in children aged 3–10 years (2nd ed.): a review of the literature on parent-training programmes and child behaviour outcome measures*. Oxford: Health Services Research Unit, University of Oxford, 1999.

23 Sheeber LB, Johnson JH. Evaluation of a temperament-focused, parent-training programme. *J Clin Child Psychol* 1994;23:249–9.

24 Bernal ME, Klinnert MD, Schultz LA. Outcome evaluation of behavioural parent-training and client-centered parent counseling for children with conduct-problems. *J Appl Behav Anal* 1980;13:677–91.

25 Herbert M. A collaborative model of training for parents of children with disruptive behaviour disorders. *Br J Clin Psychol* 1995;34:325–42.

26 Henggeler SW, Melton GB, Brondino MJ, Scherer DG, Hanley JH. Multisystemic therapy with violent and chronic juvenile offenders and their families: the role of treatment fidelity in successful dissemination. *J Consult Clin Psychol* 1997;65:831–3.
27 Smith C. *Developing parenting programmes*. London: National Children's Bureau, 1996.
28 Parenting Education & Support Forum (www.parenting-forum.org.uk). London.

4: Cognitive behaviour therapies

RICHARD HARRINGTON

Overview

Cognitive behavioural approaches are now widely used to treat psychiatric disorders in children and adolescents.

Cognitive behaviour therapy (CBT) in young people is based on the assumption that psychiatric disorders are due in part to deficiencies in particular cognitive processes or skills.

A wide variety of procedures are included in CBT. Cognitive techniques focus on changing thinking in order to produce changes in behaviour or mood.

However, cognitive behavioural formulations also emphasise the learning process and the ways in which the child's external environment can change both cognition and behaviour.

Cognitive therapy requires active collaborative involvement by patient and therapist.

The cognitive and behavioural therapies have been used for many different types of child psychiatric disorder, but the evidence base is strongest for depression, anxiety, and conduct disorders.

CBT works best in older children and adolescents with mild or moderate problems who live in stable social contexts. It has not yet been thoroughly evaluated in children with severe disorders.

Introduction

Treatments focusing on changing children's and young people's thinking and behaviour are used increasingly widely in child and adolescent mental health practice. This involves a general move toward more focused and goal directed interventions, and is strongly supported by growing evidence that interventions of this kind work efficiently.

At the core of cognitive behavioural interventions is the notion that thinking, mood, and behaviour are intimately linked and that changes in one area lead to changes in the others.

Techniques

Cognitive behaviour therapists use a variety of different techniques when working individually with children. The choice of technique depends on many factors, including the child's developmental level, the nature of the disorder being treated, and the therapist's psychological model of the causes of the child's problems. However, most of the cognitive behaviour therapies (CBTs) have the following features in common.

Therapist stance

The stance of the cognitive behaviour therapist working with children has been described using terms such as consultant and educator.[1] The therapist is active and involved but does not have all the answers. Rather, the therapist seeks to develop a collaborative relationship that stimulates the child to think for himself or herself. There is an emphasis on the child learning through experience. Thus, as with CBT in adults, there are homework assignments in which the child carries out tasks that are agreed in the session. These are often framed as an experiment. For example, a child may feel that he or she is disliked by a friend, who will avoid the child if possible. The child and therapist may conclude that the best way of finding out is for the child to try and talk to the friend.

Assessment, goal setting, and initial formulation

The assessment aims to provide a detailed description of the presenting problem that is consistent with a cognitive behavioural formulation of the child's difficulties. The assessment should also provide information about the child's social context and about their strengths and weaknesses.

The initial interview begins with a thorough review of the presenting problems and any associated symptoms. In collaboration with the child and family, the therapist carries out a detailed analysis of what are often vaguely defined presenting complaints to generate more specific target problems. The aim is to generate a shortlist of problems that are most distressing to the child and carers and that are most amenable to treatment. Standardised measures of the child's behaviour or emotions may help in defining these problems and are often a good way of measuring change. The therapist then endeavours to identify the cognitive distortions or deficits that often accompany emotional or behavioural disorders in children. Finally, an assessment is made of the child's social context with respect to family, peer relationships, neighbourhood, and education. There should be a particular emphasis on identifying strengths within both the child and the child's family or wider social environment.

The cognitive behavioural formulation is based on information from the initial assessment. It should be a written explanation of the problem that highlights the key cognitive and behavioural factors that are thought to play a role in the onset or maintenance of the child's difficulties. It should also reflect the impact of external factors, such as family difficulties or peer problems, on the young person's views of themselves and their world.

Education and engagement of the child and family

All forms of CBT should begin with an explanation of the diagnosis and the model of treatment for the child and family. The nature of this explanation depends on the child's level of cognitive development. Young people who have developed what Piaget[2] called "formal thinking skills" can usually understand the kind of explanation of CBT that would be given to adults. Such an explanation might, for instance, include the relationship between the way a person thinks about himself and his environment, and his behaviour or feelings. Many children and young adolescents find it difficult to think about thinking, however, and require explanations that are more appropriate for their developmental stage. For example, the therapist might present to the child a story about a social situation that could have several different interpretations (for example, a stranger knocking at the door) and explore with the child the various thoughts and feelings that could occur. How would the child feel, for example, if he or she thought that the stranger looked like the murderer shown on the evening news?

Parents will often be involved in CBT programmes. For example, they can help to reinforce homework assignments. In addition, they can provide information about ongoing stresses in the child's life and about the continuation of certain symptoms that the child may be reluctant to talk about (for example, peer relationship problems and antisocial behaviour).

Problem solving

A basic ingredient of both cognitive and behavioural approaches to psychiatric disorders in children is problem solving. Although the immediate antecedents of many emotional and behavioural disorders can often be identified as specific cognitions or affects, these are usually provoked by some kind of external problem. These problems are commonly of an interpersonal nature, involving either the family or peers. Training children in problem solving helps them to deal with these external problems and provides a useful model for many cognitive behaviour procedures. Problem solving in children involves much the same steps as in adults. The child is first encouraged to identify a solvable problem and then to generate as many potential solutions to it as possible. The best solution is chosen, the steps to carry it out are identified, and the child tries it out. Finally, the whole process is evaluated.

Core cognitive techniques

At the core of most of the cognitive therapies used in young people are techniques for eliciting and monitoring cognitions and for correcting distorted conceptualisations and beliefs about the world.

At all ages there is an emphasis on *self monitoring*, that is, on charting thoughts and on recording the relationship between thoughts and other phenomena such as behaviours or recent experiences. In older adolescents cognitions can be elicited using much the same techniques as in adults. In younger children it is often necessary to use more developmentally appropriate methods.

Cognitive restructuring forms an important part of many CBT programmes. The first step is to identify the thought. The thought itself should be noted down. Next, arguments and evidence to support the thought should be considered. Then arguments and evidence that cast doubt on the thought should be identified. Finally, patients should reach a reasoned conclusion, based on the available evidence, both for and against their thinking.

Problematic thoughts are often underpinned by characteristic attitudes and assumptions about the self or about the world. Typical examples include the view that in order to be happy the patient must be liked by everyone, or that aggression is a legitimate way of dealing with interpersonal conflicts. These attitudes cannot usually be identified with the approach used to identify problem thoughts because they are not fully articulated in the patient's mind. Rather, they are implicit rules that often can only be inferred from the person's behaviour. In the later stages of therapy in older adolescents, it may be possible to encourage the patient to look for patterns in his or her reactions to situations that betray these *underlying assumptions*. These techniques may be particularly useful in preventing relapse.

Core behavioural techniques

In parallel with cognitive methods, the therapist also uses relevant behavioural techniques. *Exposure* techniques are used when the client is avoiding a feared situation, such as school. Many programmes include a system of *behavioural contingencies*, in which a system of rewards is set up to reinforce desirable behaviours. Reward systems for children usually involve the parents, but in some programmes there is an emphasis on *self reinforcement*, in which the child rewards himself or herself.

Most child psychiatric disorders are worsened by inactivity. *Activity scheduling* involves the scheduling of goal directed and enjoyable activities into the child's day. The child, therapist, and caretakers collaborate to plan the young person's activities for a day on an hour by hour basis. *Specific behavioural techniques* are also used to treat certain symptoms. For example, sleep disturbance may be reduced by sleep hygiene measures. *Relaxation training* may be useful for somatic anxiety symptoms.

Applications

The CBTs have been applied to most child psychiatric disorders. The evidence base is strongest for three forms of psychopathology, namely conduct disorders, depressive disorders, and anxiety disorders.

Conduct disorders

Cognitive behavioural programmes for young people with conduct disorder and aggression usually have a strong focus on social cognitions and interpersonal problem solving. The aim of therapy is to remedy the cognitive distortions and problem solving deficits that have been identified in empirical research. Several programmes have been developed and most have the following features in common. *Self monitoring* of behaviour enables adolescents to identify and label thoughts, emotions, and the situations in which they occur. *Social perspective taking* helps them to become aware of the intentions of others in social situations.[3] Use is made of case vignettes, role play, modelling, and feedback. For example, children might be asked to describe what is going on in a picture. *Anger control training* aims to increase awareness of the early signs of hostile arousal (for example, remembering a past grudge) and to develop techniques for self control. *Problem solving skill training* attempts to remedy the deficits in cognitive problem solving processing abilities that are often found in aggressive young people.

Depressive disorders

Many slightly different cognitive behavioural approaches have been developed for depressed children and adolescents.[4] Most programmes have the following features.

First, the therapy often begins with a session, or sessions, on *emotional recognition* and *self monitoring*. The aim is to help the young person to distinguish between different emotional states (for example, sadness and anger) and to start linking external events, thoughts, and feelings.

Second, *behavioural tasks* may be used to reinforce desired behaviours and thence to help the young person to gain control over symptoms. *Self reinforcement* is often combined with *activity scheduling*, in which the young person is encouraged to engage in a programme of constructive or pleasant activities. Patients are taught to set realistic goals, with small steps toward achieving them, and to reward themselves at each successful step along the way. At this stage, it is quite common to introduce *other behavioural techniques* to deal with some of the behavioural or vegetative symptoms of depression. For example, many depressed youngsters sleep poorly and will often be helped by simple sleep hygiene measures.

Finally, various *cognitive techniques* are used to reduce depressive cognitions. For example, adolescents may be helped to identify cognitive distortions and to challenge them using techniques such as pro–con evaluation. Techniques to reduce negative automatic thoughts, such as "focus on object", are also employed.

Anxiety disorders

The principal components of CBTs for children with anxiety disorder are learning to deal with anxiety and practising these skills in real life situations. One of the most widely used programmes is the four step coping, or FEAR, plan.[5] The acronym FEAR is derived from the following: *Feeling frightened?* (awareness of anxiety symptoms such as somatic symptoms); *Expecting bad things to happen?* (awareness of negative self-talk); *Attitudes and actions that can help* (problem solving strategies); and *Results and rewards* (rewarding for success and dealing with failure). The programme starts with sessions to help children *identify anxious feelings* and to link these to anxiety provoking situations and to somatic symptoms such as panic attacks or abdominal pain. *Relaxation training* is then taught. The next few sessions aim to help the child to *identify anxious self talk* and to correct these thoughts using positive coping thoughts. Finally, the child is helped to practise the skills learned in the first part of the programme in increasingly realistic situations. Initially, these situations may be imagined (*imaginal exposure*) but later they may involve trips out of the clinic (*in vivo exposure*) to real life settings that invoke anxiety, such as the school.

Contraindications

Although the CBTs are being applied across an increasing number of problems, there are several relative contraindications to their use.

Developmental stage

Some of the techniques that are used in CBTs require that the patient has knowledge about cognition or is able to use executive processes, or both. For example, many programmes require the child to complete homework assignments that may involve some degree of planning (for example, phoning a friend to see whether he or she is really cross). Younger children will probably find this difficult because they are less likely to plan activities before carrying them out. Similarly, a key task in some cognitive programmes is to evaluate the evidence for and against a particular belief, such as that "my friends don't want to know me". However, the ability to hold mental representations of "theory" versus "evidence" emerges only gradually during adolescence.[6] Children younger than 10 tend to ignore evidence against their beliefs. It is only by middle adolescence that most individuals develop the skill of separating theory from evidence. Developmental stage is therefore an important determinant of the best technique for the child. As a general rule, older children and adolescents respond better to cognitive treatments than do younger children.[7] Different techniques may therefore need to be applied to children of different ages. Pre-adolescent children may need behavioural procedures or simple cognitive techniques such as self instruction training. Adolescents are more likely to benefit from cognitive techniques such as changing automatic thoughts.

Severity of disorder

One of the criticisms that is levelled at the CBTs is that they may not be effective in the most severe cases of disorder. Several researchers are now starting to address this issue, and CBT has been used, for example, as part of treatment programmes for very severe cases of conduct disorder.[10] Nevertheless, it must be said that much of the research that has been conducted until now with the CBTs has been based on samples recruited from adverts or through schools. Moreover, for some conditions there is evidence that severe cases respond less well to CBT than mild cases. For instance, Jayson et al.[9] reported that increased severity of social impairment was associated with reduced response to CBT in adolescents with major depression.

Social context

Emotional and behavioural disorders in young people are deeply embedded in a social context. This has implications both for how the child's problems should best be managed and for the likely response to treatment. No treatment for the child is likely to succeed if basic needs such as adequate educational opportunities or security of family placement are not met. For instance, children who are moved frequently from one home to another are unlikely to be helped by CBT, or indeed by any other kind of psychological intervention.

Evidence base

Conduct disorder

Several randomised controlled studies have found benefits from cognitive behavioural interventions with conduct disordered or aggressive children. For example, Kazdin et al.[10] used a 20-session problem solving skills programme in psychiatric inpatient children. Compared with two control conditions, the intervention led to significant reductions in parents' and teachers' ratings of aggressive behaviour after treatment and at one-year follow up. These results were replicated in two other randomised studies of problem solving training conducted by the same research group.[11,12]

Conduct disorders are notoriously difficult to treat, and these results are therefore very encouraging. Nevertheless, several limitations need to be borne in mind.[8] First, some children with conduct disorder do not respond to CBT. Children with co-morbid diagnoses or poor peer relationships, or who come from dysfunctional families seem to be less likely to respond. Such children may do better with combination treatments such as multisystemic therapy, which seems to be effective in severely impaired patients.[13] Second, the clinical significance of the changes found in these studies is unclear.[8] Many children still have some conduct problems after treatment.

Depression

At least six randomised controlled studies of CBT have been conducted in samples of children with depressive symptoms recruited through schools.[14] The design has usually been to screen all children with a depression questionnaire and then to invite those with a high score to participate in a group intervention. In four of the trials, cognitive therapy was significantly superior to no treatment.

Encouraging results have also been obtained for clinically diagnosed cases of depressive disorder. A quantitative meta-analysis of six studies found a significant improvement in the CBT group over the comparison interventions.[15] The pooled odds ratio in an intent to treat analysis was 2·2.

Anxiety disorders

Behavioural therapy is probably a useful treatment for school refusal that is secondary to anxiety disorder. For example, Miller et al.[16] found that behavioural treatment was more effective than waiting list in decreasing children's fears. Two randomised trials from the same research programme suggested that CBT is also an effective treatment for anxiety symptoms.[17]

Conclusion

All in all, this brief review suggests that, as compared either with no treatment or with a credible psychological placebo, the CBTs are effective for a number of mental or behavioural disorders. Future research will need to establish whether they are effective in severe forms of emotional disorder and how they are best combined with other treatments for conduct disorder.

Acknowedgements

Parts of this chapter are based on Harrington RC. Cognitive behaviour therapies for children and adolescents. In: Gelder MG, Lopez-Ibor JJ, Andreasen N, eds. *New Oxford textbook of psychiatry*, vol. 2. Oxford: Oxford University Press, 2000.

References

1 Kendall PC, ed. *Child and adolescent therapy*. Cognitive-behavioural procedures. New York: Guilford, 1991.
2 Piaget J. Piaget's theory. In: Mussen PH, ed. *Carmichael's manual of child psychology*, vol 1. New York: Wiley, 1970:703–32.
3 Chandler MJ. Egocentrism and anti-social behavior: the assessment and training of social perspective-taking skills. *Dev Psychol* 1973;9:326–32.
4 Harrington RC, Wood A, Verduyn C. Clinically depressed adolescents. In: Graham P, ed. *Cognitive behaviour therapy for children and families*. Cambridge: Cambridge University Press, 1998:156–93.
5 Kendall PC, Chansky TE, Kane MT, et al. Anxiety disorders in youth. *Cognitive behavioral interventions*. Needham Heights, MA: Allyn & Bacon, 1992.
6 Kuhn D, Amsel E, O'Loughlin M. *The development of scientific thinking skills*. San Diego, CA: Academic Press, 1988.
7 Durlak JA, Fuhrman T, Lampman C. Effectiveness of cognitive-behavior therapy for maladaptive children: a meta-analysis. *Psychol Bull* 1991;110:204–14.
8 Kazdin AE. Practitioner review: psychosocial treatments for conduct disorder in children. *J Child Psychol Psychiatry* 1997;38:161–78.
9 Jayson D, Wood AJ, Kroll L, Fraser J, Harrington RC. Which depressed patients respond to cognitive-behavioral treatment? *J Am Acad Child Adolesc Psychiatry* 1998;37:35–9.
10 Kazdin AE, Esveldt-Dawson K, French NH, Unis AS. Problem-solving skills training and relationship therapy in the treatment of antisocial child behavior. *J Consult Clin Psychol* 1987;55:76–85.
11 Kazdin AE, Bass D, Siegel T, Thomas C. Cognitive-behavioural therapy and relationship therapy in the treatment of children referred for antisocial behaviour. *J Consult Clin Psychol* 1989;57:522–35.
12 Kazdin AE, Esveldt-Dawson K, French NH, Unis AS. Effects of parent managment training and problem-solving skills training combined in the treatment of antisocial child behavior. *J Am Acad Child Adolesc Psychiatry* 1987;26:416–24.
13 Henggeler SW, Melton GB, Smith LA. Family preservation using multisystemic therapy: an effective alternative to incarcerating serious juvenile offenders. *J Consult Clin Psychol* 1992;60:953–61.

14 Harrington RC, Whittaker J, Shoebridge P. Psychological treatment of depression in children and adolescents: a review of treatment research. *Br J Psychiatry* 1998; **173**:291–8.

15 Harrington R, Whittaker J, Shoebridge P, Campbell F. Systematic review of efficacy of cognitive behaviour therapies in child and adolescent depressive disorder. *BMJ* 1998;**316**:1559–63.

16 Miller LC, Barrett CL, Hampe E, Noble H. Comparison of reciprocal inhibition, psychotherapy and waiting list control for phobic children. *J Abnorm Psychol* 1972;**79**:269–79.

17 Kendall PC, Flannery-Schroeder E, Panichelli-Mindel SM, Southam-Gerow M, Henin A, Warman M. Therapy for youths with anxiety disorders: a second randomized clinical trial. *J Consult Clin Psychol* 1997;**65**:366–80.

5: Interpersonal psychotherapy for adolescent depression

ERIC FOMBONNE

Overview

Interpersonal psychotherapy (IPT) is a brief (12 sessions) and focused psychotherapy that is suitable for the treatment of adolescent depression. A manual is available but specific training of the therapist is required.

IPT makes no assumption about the causes or mechanisms of depression.

Treatment aims to reduce depressive symptoms and improve social functioning.

In the initial phase, psychoeducation on depression is used and all current relationships of the patients are explored. A focus of treatment is chosen depending on the predicament of the patient.

In the middle and termination phases of treatment the therapist helps the patient to address communication difficulties, improve or dissolve problematic relationships, grieve for lost ones, adjust to new social roles, and improve social networks.

The therapist focuses on the here and now throughout treatment, and makes connections between the onset or offset of depressive symptoms in relation to social events experienced by the patient.

As in many adult studies, in recent randomised studies conducted in adolescents IPT has been shown to reduce depressive symptoms and improve social functioning, and to be more effective than routine care and as effective as cognitive behaviour therapy.

Introduction

Interpersonal psychotherapy (IPT) was first developed during the mid-1960s as a brief, time limited psychotherapy for depressed adults.[1,2] Since then modifications to IPT have been developed to treat specific psychiatric conditions, such as eating disorders,[3,4] drug addiction,[5] late depression[6] and antepartum depression,[7] or to address specific situations such as marital problems, or patients with HIV or bipolar illness.[2,8] A downward extension for adolescents (IPT for adolescents [IPT-A]) with major depression has also been developed by the Columbia Group.[9,10]

IPT-A is a time limited treatment for adolescents with major depression, which is suitable for those aged 12–18 years with the exception of those with high suicidal risk, psychotic depression, or bipolar disorder. IPT-A is structured around 12 weekly sessions, and therefore lasts for about three months. Unlike most supportive, expressive forms of psychotherapy that are often used to treat depressed adolescents and that are not standardised, a treatment manual is available for IPT-A[10] and specific training of the therapist is required. The specific goals of IPT-A are to alleviate depressive symptoms and to improve interpersonal functioning of the depressed adolescent. Thus, IPT-A is a symptom orientated, highly focused intervention.

Conceptual background of interpersonal psychotherapy for adolescents

The development of IPT was inspired by the work of influential theoreticians such as Meyer, Sullivan, and Bowlby, who emphasised the roles of attachment and relationship disturbances in the onset of psychiatric disorder. Empirically, the association between stress, life events and loss of social attachments, and the onset, course and outcome of adult depression has been supported in many studies. Clinical studies of depressed adults have also consistently shown the importance of social impairment in both acutely depressed and recovered patients, whereas intimacy and social support have been shown to be protective and to increase resilience in the face of adversity.[1]

IPT is not tied to a particular aetiological model of depression and recognises that depression can occur through different pathways in which biological, psychological, genetic, and social factors act in various combinations. However, depression, irrespective of its particular cause, occurs in a social and interpersonal context that influences its onset, course, and outcome. IPT aims to impact on current depressive symptomatology and social functioning but, because IPT is a therapeutic intervention of low intensity with a focus on the *current* depressive episode, no attempt is made to address character pathology or personality.

Role of the therapist in interpersonal psychotherapy for adolescents

The therapist is the patient's advocate and does not remain neutral. The therapist must speak for the patient, explain his or her problems, and find practical solutions to them. The therapist must be active and not passive, engaging in various activities of liaison with the family and the school when the need arises. Similarly, the therapist may involve the parents at the end of some sessions, with the agreement of the patient, in order to facilitate communication between therapist, patient, and family. The focus is on the "here and now" of the patient's network of relationships and not on past experiences.

Techniques used in interpersonal psychotherapy for adolescents

A wide array of techniques is used in IPT-A that may be tailored to the particular patient's problems.

Education is an important initial component of IPT-A and consists of providing information about depression, its symptoms, its nature, and its outcome to both patients and significant others. This educative component is seen as an important initial step in the therapy.

Exploratory techniques of a non-directive kind are used by the therapist to acknowledge the patient's difficulties in a supportive way, and to convey to the patient a sense of being accepted and understood.

Clarification is used to help the patient recognise, understand and communicate feelings, for example making links between behaviours, feelings and thoughts, but as they occur in a relational context that is meaningful to the patient. Clarification of expectations within specific relationships is also used, particularly for adolescents whose roles are changing under various developmental pressures that require the adolescent and his or her relatives to adapt their own expectations in a reciprocal and flexible manner.

Problem solving can be used to help the patient to address specific problem areas and conflicts, for instance by helping the patient to generate alternative solutions.

Encouragement of affect is a commonly used technique that aims to facilitate expression, understanding, and management of feelings by adolescents. It may consist of facilitating the acceptance of painful affects or encouraging the development of new ones.

Enhancement in *communication skills* is obtained using various techniques, including *role play* within therapeutic sessions or *social skills training* in adolescents with deficient interpersonal skills. Communication analysis is used in sessions in which the script of problematic relationships is reviewed with the patient in order to detect incorrect assumptions in the relationship, or ambiguous or paradoxical features of non-verbal communication. Straightforward *behavioural change* techniques are used sparingly in role play sequences, or in helping the patient to generate solutions to actual problems (decision analysis). To a large extent, the implementation of behavioural measures remains non-directive.

Thus, the therapeutic stance and most of the therapeutic techniques used in IPT-A do not differ from those in other forms of

Table 5.1 Interpersonal psychotherapy for adolescents, cognitive behaviour therapy, and psychodynamic therapy

	IPT-A	CBT	Psychodynamic therapy
Depression	Primary, multifactorial	Due to dysfunctional beliefs and distorted cognitive style	Derives from guilt, anger, hostility
Focus	Here and now; on actual relationships	Here and now; on cognitions and belief systems	Past experiences; on intrapsychic processes
Goals	Symptom relief	Symptom relief	Personality change
Time frame	Time limited	Time limited	Longer term
Therapist	Active, supportive	Active, supportive	Neutral; not intervening
Technique	No interpretation of therapeutic relation; no homework, within-session practice	No interpretation of therapeutic relation; task assignment	Transference is interpreted; no active techniques

CBT, cognitive behaviour therapy; IPT-A, Interpersonal psychotherapy for adolescents.

psychotherapies. Where IPT-A differs from other interventions is in the strategies used to apply the therapeutic stance and techniques for specific tasks, and in the constant focus on the interpersonal context. Similarities and differences between IPT-A and two other common forms of individual therapy are summarised in Table 5.1.

Outline of interpersonal psychotherapy for adolescents

IPT-A is conveniently divided into an initial phase (sessions 1–4), a middle phase (sessions 5–8) and a termination phase (sessions 9–12), although some flexibility is needed regarding these time divisions.

Initial phase

The goals of sessions 1–4 are summarised in Box 5.1. The first major objective is to educate the adolescent patient as to what depression is, how it affects their life, and how it impinges on their relationships with significant others. It is useful to start the treatment by reviewing the depressive symptomatology reported by the patient and to assess the severity of each symptom. Diagnosing depression as a disorder, or giving it a name, allows the patient and family to distance themselves from the disorder and helps to communicate its effects. It is also useful to give the patient a limited sick role (i.e. reducing the amount of homework or home chores that the patient would ordinarily be expected to do). Other issues need to be carefully assessed, such as the occurrence of co-morbid psychiatric disorders (in particular substance abuse).[11] The therapist will need to evaluate the possibility of using antidepressant medication in selected cases, and to address issues regarding school attendance or underachievement.

Box 5.1 Goals of the initial phase (sessions 1–4) of interpersonal psychotherapy for adolescents (IPT-A)

Deal with depression:
  Review depressive symptoms
  Give the syndrome a name
  Educate about depression (child and parent)
  Give to the patient a limited sick role
  Evaluate other aspects.

Relate depression to interpersonal context:
  Construct an inventory of relationships
  Identify expectations, satisfying and unsatisfying aspects, and changes that patient wants to make, among other components.

Identify problem areas:
  Determine problem area related to current depression
  Treatment goals (i.e. which aspects of which relationships are related to depression and might be changed).

Assess suitability of patient for IPT-A

Set a treatment contract:
  Outline your understanding of the problem(s)
  Agree on treatment goals
  Discuss practical issues.

The second goal is to establish links between the depressive symptoms and the interpersonal context in which they occur. An inventory of relationships is made, which provides a panoramic view of the network of relationships that are significant for the patient. Those relationships that are dysfunctional and those that are protective and supportive are identified in order to pinpoint communication problems and clarify expectations within and from relationships. This helps the patient to decide which changes he or she wants to make in specific relationships. When constructing the interpersonal inventory, the therapist constantly makes links between interpersonal events and fluctuations in depressive symptomatology, which help to understand the depression as influenced by the interpersonal context. This inventory of relationships also helps the therapist to identify one or two key problem areas that will be the focus of the rest of the treatment. Agreement must be reached between the therapist and the patient on what are the key problem areas and the therapist must ensure that reasonable family support is available to the patient when embarking on psychotherapy. If the family is too dysfunctional, it might well be that other forms of intervention would take precedence over individual treatment (i.e. inpatient admission or involvement of social services).

When the initial phase is completed, a treatment contract must be set between the therapist and the patient that renders explicit the understanding of the current problems and the specific treatment goals to both patient and parents. A discussion of practical issues regarding the time and frequency of sessions, what to do about missed sessions, issues of confidentiality, and ways in which the therapist may handle suicidal risk must then be held openly.

Middle phase

One or two problem areas are selected from those listed in Box 5.2 as the focus of the middle phase of IPT-A. The congruence between these problem areas and the normal challenges that occur during adolescent development is striking.

Box 5.2 Problem areas in the middle phase of interpersonal psychotherapy for adolescents

Grief
Role disputes
Role transitions
Interpersonal deficits
Single parent family.

The first area, namely *grief*, is selected when the depression relates to a form of distorted, delayed, or chronic grief following the loss of a loved figure. It will aim at helping the adolescent to acknowledge the loss and the feelings of abandonment that accompany it, to re-evaluate the pluses and minuses of the lost relationship, and to appraise the remaining relationships and social networks available to him or her more realistically.

Role disputes is an area selected for conflictual relationships, typically between adolescent and parents or a boyfriend or girlfriend, when a link between these conflicts and depressive symptomatology is found. The aims are to open new negotiations between the involved parties, to acknowledge role changes and modify expectations within the relationships, and to modify communication patterns.

The third problem area, *role transitions*, is selected when the depressive symptoms relate to difficulties in changing roles within the developmental process, either because the parents do not accept new roles in the adolescent or because the adolescent has his or her own difficulties in coping with new demands and expectations. This typically occurs with the passage from group to dyadic relationships, with the emergence of intimate sexual relationships, with key normative transitions such as leaving home or planning a career, and with unforeseen circumstances such as adolescent pregnancy.

The fourth problem area, namely *interpersonal deficits*, is selected when the onset and maintenance of depressive symptoms in the adolescent is linked to a lack of interpersonal skills and social isolation that can be improved using communication analysis and direct teaching of relevant social skills.

The fifth and final problem area, namely *single parent family*, was added specifically for the adolescent version of IPT, recognising the fact that, currently, many adolescents live within single parent families or have had to deal with the departure of one of their parents from their home. This area will help to address feelings of loss and rejection, to clarify expectations from the relationship with the parent who left, to negotiate harmonious and working relationships with custodial parents, and to accept the permanence of the separation between the parents.

Termination phase

The last four sessions are devoted to reviewing progress and changes that were accomplished in therapy, and to assessing residual symptoms of depression. An explicit discussion of the termination before the last session should be initiated by the therapist, and an acknowledgment of the difficulties of terminating the therapeutic relationship should be facilitated. This may be used to promote the recognition of independent competence in the adolescent by the therapist. The issue of relapse or future depressive recurrence should also be addressed, and the adolescent should by then have a clear knowledge of which symptoms to monitor and how to recognise the imminence of a relapse. A plan that ensures that proper assistance will be available should be rehearsed. Co-morbid psychiatric disorders that were not the focus of IPT-A can also be addressed subsequently with specific interventions.

Involving parents and the school

As mentioned for the initial phase, parents will be involved specifically at the beginning of the treatment to ensure their participation in the diagnostic assessment and to improve their own understanding and knowledge of depression, its presentation, its outcome, and its treatment. The parents are also part of the initial phase when a specific treatment contract is set between the therapist and the adolescent patient. Parents should be knowledgeable about the practical goals of the treatment and what will be left untouched by the therapist. Parents must also be informed about issues both of confidentiality and of communication between the therapist and themselves if circumstances indicate this (for example, suicidal risk). The parents will also be involved in the middle phase when the therapist works with the adolescent on specific targets. This may take the form of the therapist spending some time with the adolescent and the parents at the end of sessions to discuss issues relevant to family life that are considered to impinge on treatment progress.

Liaison with the school is also a key component of intervention, and the therapist, or a professional colleague from the same team, may have to explain the depression in the adolescent who has failed to attend or to achieve at school (educational aspect). Furthermore, they may have to negotiate with the school the practical steps that can be taken to facilitate re-attendance of the patient who has been refusing to go to school, and to increase the likelihood of satisfactory achievement when recovery is on its way (intervention aspect).

Evidence for the efficacy of interpersonal psychotherapy

Several well designed randomised controlled trials have been conducted with IPT both in the treatment of acute depression in adults and in maintenance.[2] In the early 1970s acute treatment studies showed that IPT and tricyclic antidepressant intervention had roughly equal efficacy versus control conditions in the treatment of acute depression, with an improved effect for the combination of drug and psychotherapy.[12] Interestingly, although antidepressant medication had a slightly quicker effect in alleviating symptoms, IPT appeared to be associated with better psychosocial functioning at follow up. In a 16 week treatment of 250 depressed adults, a US National Institute of Mental Health study confirmed that cognitive behaviour therapy, IPT, and imipramine had similar effects over control conditions, with a trend however toward a superiority of IPT over CBT in the most severe cases.[13] In a meta-analysis, combined pharmacotherapy and psychotherapy was found to produce better results when the major depression is severe.[14] Similarly, the response to IPT was poorer among adult depressives with abnormal sleep profiles, indicating greater neurobiological disturbance.[15] The limited research evidence on the cost effectiveness of psychotherapy and pharmacotherapy suggests slight superiority of pharmacotherapy,[16] but data thus far are too scarce to draw even preliminary conclusions on this issue.

IPT has also been tested as a maintenance treatment to prevent further relapse in adults. It was shown to improve social functioning after six months of treatment, and the combination of IPT with drug treatment appeared to carry the best effect.[12,17] Broadly similar results were found in a three year maintenance trial comparing high dose imipramine with a low frequency form of IPT (one session per month), in which the latter was superior to placebo and more efficacious in combination with drug treatment.[18] The same pattern of better maintenance with combined nortriptyline and IPT over single modality treatments has been demonstrated for older depressives.[6]

Because IPT-A was developed recently, there are fewer systematic studies investigating its efficacy.[11,19] In one open trial, the Columbia University group described pre- and post-treatment differences in a group of 14 adolescents with a mean age of 15·5 years.[20] At post-treatment, 90% of this small sample had recovered from their major depression, and exhibited a significant decrease over time in depressive rating scales, including the Beck Depression Inventory and the Hamilton Rating Scale for Depression. Improvement was noted in several areas of social functioning. A one year follow up study conducted in 10 patients in that initial sample showed that treatment gains had been maintained.[21] Mufson et al.[22] then completed a randomised clinical trial assessing the efficacy of IPT-A in a controlled experiment. In that study, 48 adolescents aged 12–18 years who met criteria for major depression were randomly assigned to either 12 weekly sessions of IPT-A or clinical monitoring. A significantly greater proportion of subjects (88% versus 46%) completed the IPT-A treatment as compared with the control condition. A significantly greater proportion (75%) of IPT-A treated patients met recovery criteria as compared with the control group (46%), and their social functioning was also better. These findings support the efficacy of IPT-A in treating acutely depressed adolescents.

Another study compared the efficacy of CBT and IPT in 71 depressed adolescents randomly assigned to one of three groups: CBT, IPT, or waiting list.[23] Pretreatment, post-treatment, and three month follow up measures suggested that IPT and CBT significantly reduced depressive symptoms as compared with the waiting list condition. IPT was superior to waiting list in increasing self esteem and social adaptation. Further analyses suggested that 82% of adolescents in the IPT group and 59% of those in the CBT group were functional after treatment, thereby providing some evidence that IPT was associated with better social functioning outcomes than alternative brief therapies. Ongoing controlled studies are being conducted to compare the efficacy of IPT with that of antidepressant drugs, and the efficacy of IPT administered in group formats in school settings is also being investigated.

Conclusion

IPT is a brief treatment (12 sessions) that is available for treatment of adolescent depression. A manual is available but specific training of the therapist in IPT is mandatory. The treatment approach focuses on the "here and now" and on the interpersonal context of the depressed adolescent, and its goals are to achieve rapid alleviation of depressive symptoms and improvement in social functioning. Adult studies have consistently shown the efficacy of IPT as a psychotherapeutic treatment modality for acute depression and relapse prevention, and recent studies conducted in adolescent patients have demonstrated the efficacy of IPT in treating acute depressive episodes.

References

1   Klerman GL, Weissman MM, Rounsaville BJ, Chevron ES, eds. *Interpersonal psychotherapy for depression.* New York: Basic Books, 1984.
2   Weissman MM, Markowitz JC. Interpersonal psychotherapy. *Arch Gen Psychiatry* 1994;**51**:599–606.
3   Fairburn C, Jones R, Peveler R, *et al*. Three psychological treatments for bulimia nervosa: a comparative trial. *Arch Gen Psychiatry* 1991;**48**:463–9.
4   Fairburn C, Jones R, Peveler R, Hope R, O'Connor M. Psychotherapy and bulimia nervosa: longer-term effects of interpersonal psychotherapy, behavior therapy, and cognitive behavior therapy. *Arch Gen Psychiatry* 1993;**50**:419–28.
5   Carroll KM, Rounsaville BJ, Gawin FH. A comparative trial of psychotherapies for ambulatory cocaine abusers: relapse prevention and interpersonal psychotherapy. *Am J Drug Alcohol Abuse* 1991;**17**:229–47.
6   Reynolds C, Frank E, Perel J, *et al*. Nortriptyline and interpersonal psychotherapy as maintenance therapies for recurrent major depression. *JAMA* 1999;**281**:39–45.
7   Spinelli M. Interpersonal psychotherapy for depressed antepartum women: a pilot study. *Am J Psychiatry* 1997;**154**:1028–30.
8   Klerman GL, Weissman MM, eds. *New applications of interpersonal psychotherapy.* Washington, DC: American Psychiatric Press, 1993.
9   Moreau D, Mufson L, Weissman MM, Klerman GL. Interpersonal psychotherapy for adolescent depression: description of modification and preliminary application. *J Am Acad Child Adolesc Psychiatry* 1991;**30**:642–51.
10 Mufson L, Moreau D, Weissman W, Klerman G. *Interpersonal psychotherapy for depressed adolescents.* New York: Guilford Press, 1993.
11 Fombonne E. The management of depression in children and adolescents. In: Checkley S, ed. *Handbook on the management of depression.* Oxford: Blackwell Publications, 1998:345–63.
12 Klerman GL, DiMascio A, Weissman MM, Prusoff BA, Paykel ES. Treatment of depression by drugs and psychotherapy. *Am J Psychiatry* 1974;**131**:186–91.
13 Elkin I, Shea MT, Watkins JT, *et al*. National Institute of Mental Health Treatment of Depression Collaborative Research Program: general effectiveness of treatments. *Arch Gen Psychiatry* 1989;**46**:971–82.
14 Thase M, Greenhouse J, Frank E, *et al*. Treatment of major depression with psychotherapy or psychotherapy-pharmacotherapy combinations. *Arch Gen Psychiatry* 1997;**54**:1009–15.
15 Thase M, Buysse D, Frank E, *et al*. Which depressed patients will respond to interpersonal psychotherapy? The role of abnormal EEG sleep profiles. *Am J Psychiatry* 1997;**154**:502–9.
16 Lave J, Frank R, Schulberg HC, Kamlet MS. Cost-effectiveness of treatments for major depression in primary care practice. *Arch Gen Psychiatry* 1998;**55**:645–51.

17   Weissman MM, Prusoff BA, DiMascio A, Neu C, Goklaney M, Klerman GL. The efficacy of drugs and psychotherapy in the treatment of acute depressive episodes. *Am J Psychiatry* 1979;**136**:555–8.
18   Frank E, Kupfer DJ, Wagner EF, McEachran AB, Cornes C. Efficacy of interpersonal psychotherapy as a maintenance treatment of recurrent depression: contributing factors. *Arch Gen Psychiatry* 1991;**48**:1053–9.
19   American Academy of Child and Adolescent Psychiatry. Practice parameters for the assessment and treatment of children and adolescent with depressive disorders. *J Am Acad Child Adolesc Psychiatry* 1998;**37(suppl)**:63S–83S.
20   Mufson L, Moreau D, Weissman MM, Wickramaratne P, Martin J, Samoilov A. Modification of interpersonal psychotherapy with depressed adolescents (IPT-A): phase I and II studies. *J Am Acad Child Adolesc Psychiatry* 1994;**33**:695–705.
21   Mufson L, Fairbanks J. Interpersonal psychotherapy for depressed adolescents: a one-year naturalistic follow-up study. *J Am Acad Child Adolesc Psychiatry* 1996;**35**: 1145–55.
22   Mufson L, Weissman M, Moreau D, Garfinkel R. Efficacy of interpersonal psychotherapy for depressed adolescents. *Arch Gen Psychiatry* 1999;**56**:573–9.
23   Rossello J, Bernal G. The efficacy of cognitive-behavioral and interpersonal treatments for depression in Puerto Rican adolescents. *J Consult Clin Psychol* 1999; **67**:734–45.

6: Non-directive individual work with children

JUDITH TROWELL

Overview

Non-directive individual psychotherapy traditionally appeared to be indicated
  for extremely emotionally disturbed young children, for those living with sick
  family members, or for older adolescents.
The treatment is being offered increasingly to abused or fostered children and
  in special schools for emotionally disturbed children.
Children in other personal predicaments may benefit, or their parents may do so.
Treatment may include play therapy, brief or long-term psychodynamic therapy,
  or creative art therapies.
Individual work can helpfully explore early and current child relationships and
  attachment issues.
It aims to help young people reduce distress, improve symptoms, and promote
  change.
Multiple case studies have described improvements in a number of children,
  but study designs preclude demonstration of efficacy.

Introduction

Individual work can benefit many children and young people seen in
Child and Adolescent Mental Health Services who have difficulties,
and can be helpful in situations where there are family problems.
However, the assessment process is crucial. If the problem is family
based or if there is intense pressure to view the child as the problem,
then there is a need to proceed with caution; labelling the child as the
patient may be quite damaging. In adolescence, this process can
happen all too easily. Normal adolescent turmoil can impose stress on
a vulnerable family or marriage,[1] and adolescents can then be seen as
a problem in the absence of psychiatric disorder. Nevertheless, some
of these young people, despite no formal diagnosis, can benefit from
individual help to assist in the ordinary process of separation and
individuation from a family in disarray. It is important in these cases
to be clear to the individual, the family, and the worker that this is the
task and purpose of the work.

This chapter first outlines indications for individual work, with case examples. Then, different modes of therapy, including play therapy, brief therapy, long-term therapy, and creative arts therapies, are described. Finally, the advantages of individual work and its effectiveness, together with some contraindications, are summarised.

Indications for individual work

When assessing cases it is important to have in mind a variety of therapeutic options. These may range from the opinion that the child is internally healthy and is coping in an adverse family and social setting, to the view that the child is profoundly damaged and needs intensive treatment in a residential setting. It is essential not to ignore the needs of the family, the alternative care givers, and the professional network, and an essential part of the assessment is unravelling all of these factors. When might one recommend individual psychodynamic therapy for a child? Martin and Knight[2] proposed three main areas in which individual psychodynamic therapy may be appropriate, and others have since added to these.[3-5] The following have been suggested.

Extremely disturbed young children

Martin and Knight[2] stated that in some cases – whatever trauma has been inflicted on the child and after the family has made considerable improvements – it is still possible for some children to be left with internal representational models that are so bizarre and so out of reach of normal family interaction that only individual psychodynamic therapy or work can reach them. The aim of this work is to access the inaccessible, and so allow the child to be free to relate to and use the emotional experiences that are now on offer by the family.

Where a family system is actively and crucially engaged in supporting a very sick member and there is active resistance to change

At a particular point around puberty, the child is beginning to separate. In these situations, helping the child to establish their own identity, to test out reality, and to free them from guilt about their role in the dilemma can be vital in enabling them to survive emotionally intact.

Older adolescents aged 16–20 years – a period of transition

Some families may find it all but impossible to allow the child to move off. Often, a brief focused individual psychotherapeutic input can be helpful.

Additional indications for individual work

The three categories described above have now been supplemented to include additional ones. This may be because cases currently referred to child and family mental health teams are more complex, and services are expected to find ways to intervene helpfully for them. Some clinicians have offered individual therapy, and sometimes increasingly positively so in the light of experience.

Abused children

Some clinicians see large numbers of children in whom abuse has occurred or is still taking place, including physical, emotional or sexual abuse, or neglect. Some of these children are referred at the time of abuse, whereas others are referred years later when problems are arising in their foster or adoptive placement.

Abused children in whom all of the necessary protective steps have been taken may have been subjected to prolonged abuse, generally sexual or emotional. Family work and group work can be helpful, but there are a number of profoundly damaged, emotionally fragmented children who are unable to function at school or in interpersonal relationships. Sometimes, the actual abuse may not have been prolonged, but a single instance of abuse or rape may reveal a "victimee" – a very vulnerable child, who is deprived and neglected – where it appears that the abuse has brought the child to someone's attention.[6]

Our specialist Child and Adolescent Mental Health Service team has become increasingly aware of the large numbers of *children in special schools for emotionally and behaviourally disturbed or learning disabled children* who have been or are still being subjected to abuse (it may be sexual). This may only emerge within the context of the privacy and trust that a child is offered in individual work.

Fostered or adopted children (see example below)

Many referrals involve children in whom the second, third, or fourth foster placement is breaking down; when the adoptive family is considering seeking dissolution of the adoption; or when a reconstituted family cannot integrate a particular child. When family work cannot offer enough because the individual child is so internally damaged, psychodynamic therapy may help.[7]

Our team now receives referrals in which such children are back in some form of institutional care and it is recognised they cannot cope with the stress of family life and need preparation before a fresh attempt can be made to place them.

Chronic illness

Psychodynamic therapy can help some children with chronic physical illness such as diabetes, cystic fibrosis, or muscular dystrophy, particularly around puberty. Terminally ill children, for example those in bone marrow transplant units or renal transplant units, may also be helped.

Developmental disorders

Some children and young people with Asperger's syndrome or other autistic spectrum disorder may respond well to non-directive work. This does not attempt to cure the disorder but does focus on helping the individual to accept their difficulties and maximise their potential.

Counselling of children under five and parent–infant psychotherapy

There have been increased referrals in both of these areas to the specialist services in recent years. Families may be seen together in mother and child therapy, or there may be brief work with the parents and child. The difficulties often present as sleep problems, feeding problems, temper tantrums, or more general behavioural problems, including sibling rivalry and enuresis or encopresis. Often, the problem has become entrenched and self perpetuating, and the work must focus on the parents' or carers' past experiences while freeing the child to be viewed as such, rather than as a problem.

The transition into adolescence

Individual work with adolescents may be brief (the young people's counselling model) or may be longer term for problems such as depression, eating disorder, identity and gender identity problems, self harm, school and relationship problems, or conduct and oppositional defiant disorder.[8]

Life events

Finally, and less dramatically, there is a group of children that deserves our attention. These are the children who are probably already vulnerable but coping and who, when confronted with a life event (for example, the death of a parent, a parent with mental illness, domestic violence, alcohol and substance abuse, and in some cases of divorce), cease to be able to maintain their fragile functioning and need individual help.

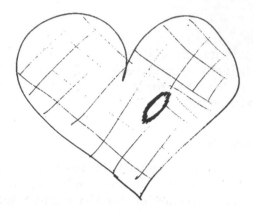

Children and young people can become distressed, confused, and depressed by life's adversities. This picture was drawn by a child aged eight in contested adoption. "All my love is for John and Mary (prospective adopters), but there'll always be a little bit in the middle for my born-to Mum"

Clinical examples

Clinical examples can illustrate the core assessment (with the wider assessment not reported). Richard and William, described below, were each (separately) referred for help with foster placements.

Case example 1

Background

Our clinic social worker had been consulting at a social services department for some time about their case management. A particular case arose that involved a foster child placed with specialist foster parents, and there was a question of his future placement. The clinic social worker and I met the local authority social worker and foster parents. I was asked to see the foster child to consider the most appropriate placement. There was also the possibility of a court hearing because his natural mother was planning to apply for revocation of the care order.

Assessment

I saw Richard, aged nine years, twice. On the first occasion he said very little, but at the end of the session he drew a milk float with a compartment for bread, eggs and cheese. I suggested that, possibly, he would like to be like the milk float, with everything he needed on board so that he didn't need anyone – he could look after himself. At the next session, Richard picked up the milk float drawing and spent the time talking about the events in his life: how his father had punched Mum, him and his brother, and he didn't know where his father was; and how Mum used to go out, leaving him and his brother in the flat. He described the heater tipping over, the fire, and how he managed to climb out of the window. He tried to pull his brother out and couldn't; he went to get someone and told his brother to get a chair to climb on. His brother died in the fire. Richard talked about his mother, whom he saw occasionally, and how he missed her and would like to be able to live with her, but he knew it was no good. Often she said she was coming to see him and then didn't turn up; she said she could do things, take him places, and then forgot. He wanted to stay with the new family – he liked it there, he liked them, and he liked the school and cubs.

He was very sad, very realistic, and despairing about his mother. My special concern was a nightmare he described of a violent fire and him burning in a cauldron, and his complete lack of apparent anger about his parents. He was burdened by the guilt of his brother's death.

Outcome

The clinic social worker and I met with the foster father, foster mother, and the local authority social worker. Richard's wish to remain in foster care was considered and some of the possible problems that might arise were aired. It seemed to me that Richard's wish was appropriate. His foster parents were likely to be the most suitable placement and so should be endorsed. His mother did not attend the court hearing for the revocation of the care order, and so Richard remained with the foster carers.

Case example 2

Background

The same foster parents requested an assessment of William, another foster child. Social services were planning to place the child with prospective adoptive parents, and his current foster parents were very concerned. They were also saying that they were not certain they could keep him in their home for much longer. He was seen as a provocative child who needled children until they lashed out at him and then he hit out. Alternatively, he just attacked other children randomly.

William was six years old; his entire life had consisted of change and moves from one care giver to another.

William's mother was the daughter of a family well known to the caring professionals. Her own mother had a history of heavy drinking and her father, a semi-invalid, also drank. There was violent discord in the home. She was one of seven children, and her brothers had drink problems and a sister had tuberculosis. She was known to be a heavy drinker and to have a history of drug abuse. William's father was believed to be a publican living in Essex. William's mother and this man had a violent, intermittent relationship.

William's mother had considered asking for him to be adopted while she was pregnant but then changed her mind. She kept the baby, but her mother looked after William until he was nearly two years old. This "looking after" consisted of a network of caregivers, maternal grandmother, and the four sisters and their children, with William moving from one to another.

William's mother took more interest in him when she was given a flat, but she was pregnant again. The second child was premature and went into a special care baby unit. She did not visit the baby and avoided screening of herself and William for tuberculosis. Under threat of an emergency protection order, she took the baby home. One month later, the baby died a "cot death". The next day, William took an overdose of his aunt's tuberculosis medication and was admitted to hospital overnight.

William continued to be cared for by mother, grandmother, and aunts. He was accommodated by social services when his grandmother arrived at nursery to collect him, drunk and unable to cope. He returned to his mother, and for about six months his life was more settled, but then she went off again to his father for long periods, leaving William once more in the care of the family circle.

William was received into care when his aunt contacted the school saying that she could no longer accept responsibility for him. William's mother was not around and admitted that she could not provide William with a home. William was collected by a social worker on an emergency protection order from school.

William was placed in a children's home and then moved to a foster home. Contact with his mother was minimal after that. Since then, she had agreed to work toward terminating her relationship with William, knowing that she could not provide him with a home to meet his needs.

The children's home report stated that William was domineering and aggressive, but also an appealing and loveable boy. The most difficult aspect of William to handle was the way in which he could drive people to distraction. He had an ability to "wind people up" that was stressed by staff in their report. He also had problems with a lifestyle involving irregular routines, and his school attending had been erratic.

Assessment

The clinic social worker and I met first with William's foster parents, who were rather tense and uncertain. They were very concerned about William and were doing their best for him, but they were also very worried by the effect he was having on their family life. William's aggression was difficult to control, but more difficult than that was something unreachable about William that left them feeling useless, frustrated, and angry. In particular, the foster father felt that they could not continue with William because he was somehow disrupting and damaging their family.

William was seen twice by me. The first thing to strike me was what an appealing and attractive boy he was, with a mop of red hair and a delightful smile. He was a good size for his age and seemed relaxed about staying with me when his foster mother introduced us. He took a ball and bounced it around the room gently at first, but soon I had to protect the pictures and plants. He flitted around the room unable to settle and played in a restless way, but it also made me feel uncomfortable somehow – nothing was good enough or of interest to him. He did not speak spontaneously. When I asked about his current life he answered briefly, but when I asked about before that he did not reply – and drew Superman. I said it looked as though he wished that he or I could be Superman and sort everything out. The only moment of eye contact was then, when he agreed. I asked about his mother and father. He had seen his mother recently but never saw his father. He turned abruptly and wouldn't say any more. I wondered whether it was too painful; "No," he said, "too sad."

He spent the rest of the time restlessly wandering round the room, picking up anything and everything and asking whether he could take it home. I explained that he could not. Ten minutes early he wanted to go. I agreed and took him to his foster mother. I was left feeling hopeless and despairing, but also relieved that he had gone. There had been something very irritating and aggravating about him, but in spite of this I felt that I had made no real contact with him.

On the second occasion he had his lunchbox with him, which he reluctantly left with his foster mother. He came quite easily with me and remembered the way to the room.

He picked over the toys in a desultory way. I had kept his drawing; he looked and said "Superman, Super William". He laughed in an unpleasant way. He found the animals and took a small lamb, discarded it, and said he was hungry. I suggested that perhaps the lamb needed caring for – feeding. He hunted for a wolf; when there wasn't one, he threw the animals away.

He took the dolls and placed a baby doll firmly in a male doll's arm and another doll was placed precariously in a female doll's arms. He took another female doll, peered up her skirt, ripped off her clothes, tore at the body, and snapped off a foot. I said he was showing me how angry he felt, particularly with women. He said he was full up with anger.

He found the paints and wanted to paint, not on the paper but on the tabletop and two of the model toys; swirls of black and red by now

73

were everywhere. That looks like blood, he pronounced gleefully. Then it was black, black everywhere – the table, the sink, him, and me. I was on my toes trying to contain the flow of blackness. When I said firmly that that was enough, I didn't encounter the defiance I expected. He accepted what I said and stood quite passively holding out his hands to be washed and dried. Once clean, he was out of the door, stating "I'm going to eat my lunch".

I found it difficult being in the room with this boy. It was a relief that he had gone early again. He was an attractive boy, who elicited warmth and concern, but within moments this froze. His contempt and denigration were insidious but very powerful, so that for a while I found it difficult to sort out what was going on. His violent sadistic rage and destructiveness were more obvious.

I did not feel that an ordinary family could handle the intense and conflictual feelings that William provoked, and that he needed a special therapeutic environment. The adults, particularly any women, would need a great deal of support in any attempt to establish a relationship with William. First appearances gave the impression of an attractive and beguiling boy, but then there followed the barrage of contempt, sabotaging everything. There was no sense of being able to make contact, and bearing this would be very difficult. Sustained periods of contact with William would be hard to bear, and adults would need periods of relief. William also had a capacity to cut off, provoking frustration and despair.

Outcome

After assessment, the recommendation was that a further placement that might break down would only increase William's violent rage and destructiveness, and for this reason a special placement was needed for him.

Types of individual non-directive work

Play therapy

Play therapy can be brief or long term. It can also focus on particular issues or be more open. Play therapy offers a child time with a sensitive, empathic, non-judgemental adult who gives them their full attention. The adult has been trained to maintain appropriate boundaries with respect to time, place, reliability and regularity, and to respond appropriately to a range of emotions from the child or young person while maintaining clear limits on physical contact. The therapist has supervision or consultation, so that their reactions to the work and their own emotional issues and agenda do not intrude or interfere.

With regard to the first case example given above, it was suggested that Richard could benefit from such play therapy. He needed to come to terms with his early experiences and his relationships now with his mother and foster carers, and to find ways of being in touch with his pain, fear, guilt, and anger. He needed to be free to engage with the foster carers, school, and friends; to develop trust and security; and to begin to hope and be creative.

Individual psychodynamic psychotherapy

Individual psychodynamic psychotherapy was recommended for William, the second case example presented above. Psychodynamic psychotherapy can be brief or long term. It can take place once weekly or more often, anything up to five times weekly, but this is very rare; more usual is two or three times weekly if intensive therapy is required. William was offered long-term therapy twice weekly. Long-term therapy is usually two years after a review at one year; rarely, it continues beyond this. The aims are similar to those of play therapy, but in addition to statements made to clarify what the child is saying or doing, there is an attempt to understand the conflicts, distress, and confusion in the child by making links between the here and now interaction, the child's play material, and what may be underlying feelings. These feelings are accessed by the therapist by using observation of the child and of the therapist's own internal state. The aim is to try to connect, through this "counter transference", with what the child may or may not be aware of consciously but which may be powerfully communicated by them in their behaviour and interaction.

It is wrong to embark on this work if those around have unrealistic expectations. The child will not emerge with a different personality, and will not necessarily become a socially conforming citizen, but may be more accepting of himself or herself, and less driven by conflicts, confusion, and inner pain.

Stages in therapy

Brief psychodynamic and long-term psychotherapy go through stages whether the therapy is 10–30 sessions, once weekly, or more long term or intensive. These stages consist of an opening introductory state; in 30 sessions, this may be the first 10 sessions. There is then a middle phase, in which there is intense involvement, the issues seem overwhelming, and the therapist feels that the individual is very troubled or disturbed and they may feel inadequate. The ending phase, the last five sessions, in which work is on separation or loss, usually results in a restoration of calm with some relief and sense of sadness. Many children and young people arrive at the ending phase in a reasonable state if all concerned have been clear about the duration of treatment and the process. If the child remains in a deeply distressed or troubled state, then the review may well recommend further work.

The more extreme the difficulties, the more work that may be required, but many young people and some children respond well to time limited work and are able to engage because they do not feel they will become trapped in never ending attendance.[9]

Creative arts therapy

Many shy and inhibited children or children with language and communication difficulties, learning difficulties, or autistic spectrum disorders can respond well to art, music, drama, or dance therapy. Through non-verbal means, patients can express themselves and at the same time gain gratification by being creative. Clinically, the results from these ways of working can be impressive.

Other non-directive models

There are a number of other non-directive interventions available, such as Gestalt therapy, and counselling has grown and spread dramatically. Counselling is often topic focused and can be offered in response to a particular problem, such as abuse, parental serious accident or illness, or after parental separation or divorce. The work is child lead and the aim is to assist the child in coming to terms with the issue. Young people tend to be offered counselling whereas children are offered play therapy, but many more articulate children receive counselling to good effect.

Advantages and strengths of individual work

Therapy with an individual child is easy to organise, requiring only the child and the worker, and so can be set up more quickly than group work. Non-directive work is child lead; the pace and the sequence of topics are determined by the child, although the worker may well have an agenda of topics for the piece of work. The work can address individual needs and can more easily keep the whole child in mind than is possible with group approaches. The work can explore early childhood relationships and current relationships, and can establish a relationship with the child based on trust and security. Attachment issues can be addressed specifically, as can issues pertaining to race, culture, sexuality, and disability. The specific meaning of separation and loss can be considered, and some young people value the privacy, for example when talking about sexual abuse or their own sexual experiences. It is possible to address urgent external world issues and then move to more internal world concerns and back to the external world in a flexible and seamless manner.

Contraindications to individual work

If the child or young person is experiencing a particular external reality, such as moving to another area, transferring to boarding school, or about to take exams, it is not appropriate to embark on an intensive piece of work. Opening up painful, distressing areas when there is no time to work them through or when the child or young person must go outside and function can be damaging. A therapeutic consultation would be the right way to proceed in such a situation.

There are also dangers if therapists find themselves out of their depth and unable to cope with a child's rage, pain, distress, or desperate need for affection.

To avoid behaving inappropriately, the therapist needs to be very clear about what is treatment and what is parenting. Suicidal young people or children experiencing abuse need to be placed somewhere safe, and be adequately parented or cared for; therapy can never replace parenting or provide monitoring. In cases that involve physical illness, acute or chronic, it is important to work with the general practitioner or paediatrician.

Effectiveness

Does this way of working provide relief and bring about change? Outcome studies of non-directive work conducted in children and young people have shown children to be improved following therapy. The author has shown prospectively that individual psychotherapy with sexually abused girls does produce improvement,[10] although methodological questions remain.[6] Fonagy and Target[11] reviewed retrospectively the 763 patients that had attended the Anna Freud Child Psychotherapy Clinic. Many improved but some did not. Those reviewers were able to indicate which children did better in once weekly work and which did better in more frequent sessions. In 1991 Barrnett et al.[12] reviewed child psychotherapy research and concluded that most studies reported until then were case studies and hence unable to demonstrate efficacy, although the children improved. They called for further methodologically sound research.

Since then many studies have been published, but most are multiple case studies[13] rather than formal outcome studies. The exceptions are in the fields of abuse, childhood depression, and eating disorders.[14]

Conclusion

Non-directive work is offered as counselling, play therapy, and individual psychodynamic psychotherapy, as well as creative arts therapy. These interventions can provide relief from distress, reduce symptoms, and promote change, but practitioners need to be encouraged to evaluate their work in a systematic manner, and to take seriously the need for an evidence base and undertake outcome studies, as have colleagues working in the field of adult therapies.

References

1 Rutter M, Graham P, Chadwick O, Yule W. Adolescent turmoil: fact or fiction? *J Child Psychol Psychiatry* 1976;**17**:35–6.
2 Martin F, Knight J. Joint interviews as part of intake procedures in a child psychiatric clinic. *J Child Psychol Psychiatry* 1962;**3**:17–26.
3 Boston M, Szur R, eds. *Psychotherapy with severely deprived children*. London: RKP, 1983.
4 Szur R, Miller S. *Extending horizons*. London: Karnac Books, 1991.
5 Jenning S. *Play therapy with children*. Oxford: Blackwell, 1993.
6 Trowell J, Kolvin I, Weeramanthri T, *et al*. Psychotherapy outcome for sexually abused girls. Psychopathological outcome and patterns of change. *Br J Psychiatry* 2002;**180**:234–47.
7 Boston M, Lush D. Further considerations of methodology for evaluating psychoanalytic psychotherapy with children: reflections in the light of research experience. *J Child Psychother* 1994;**20**:205–39.
8 Target M, Fonagy P. The efficacy of psychoanalysis for children with disruptive disorders. *J Am Acad Child Adolesc Psychiatry* 1994;**33**:45–55.
9 Messer S, Warren CS. *Models of brief psychodynamic therapy: a comparative approach in brief psychotherapy*. New York: Guilford Press, 1995.
10 Long J, Trowell J. Individual brief psychotherapy with sexually abused girls. *Psychoanal Psychother* 2001;**15**:39–59.
11 Fonagy P, Target M. Predictors of outcome in child psychoanalysis: a retrospective study of 763 cases at the Anna Freud Centre. *J Am Psychoanal Assoc* 1996;**44**:27–77.
12 Barnett RJ, Docherty J, Frommett G. Special article: a review of child psychotherapy research since 1963. *J Am Acad Child Adolesc Psychiatry* 1991;**30**:1–14.
13 Lush D, Boston M, Grainger E. Evaluation of psychoanalytic psychotherapy with children: therapists' assessments and predictions. *Psychoanal Psychother* 1991;**5**:191–234.
14 Luborsky L. *Who will benefit from psychotherapy? Predicting therapeutic outcomes*. New York: Basic Books, 1988.

7: Cognitive behavioural group work with children and adolescents

VEIRA BAILEY, BEA VICKERS

Overview

Many cognitive behaviour therapy (CBT) techniques adapt readily to use in a group setting for children of different ages, and can be incorporated into effective and enjoyable programmes for a range of problems. The group setting is ideally suited to work on social skills difficulties.

The ethos of a CBT group should be that problems can be solved and the group is an opportunity to learn skills to do this, as well as realising that one's difficulties are not unique.

Group leaders can model expression of feelings and appropriate empathising with others.

Peer modelling and ideas of other children broaden the problem solving repertoire of group members.

The research base for the efficacy and effectiveness of CBT in groups for children and adolescents has been increasing steadily over recent years.

Introduction

Cognitive behaviour therapy (CBT) has a growing evidence base across a range of disorders, although some research questions and pragmatic concerns about implementation remain.[1] Many CBT techniques adapt readily to use in a group setting, and can be modified to suit the developmental needs of young children through to adolescents if groups are appropriately age stratified.

Group work with children and adolescents can take place in a variety of settings, including schools, social service departments, and Child and Adolescent Mental Health Services (CAMHS), with frequency of groups ranging from weekly to daily depending on the intensity of the intervention. Within CAMHS settings, group interventions will usually form one component of a package of treatment.

Elements of cognitive behaviour therapy interventions used in most programmes for children and adolescents

CBT has become an umbrella term for a range of treatment techniques that can be used in different sequences and combinations. The underlying assumption in CBT is that cognitions, affect (feelings), and behaviour are closely related, and that changes in one can bring about changes in the others. Many CBT techniques are adaptable for use in groups. Indeed, many can be facilitated by the group format. The main techniques are described below, with examples of application in group settings with children and adolescents (see also Chapter 4).

Emotional (affective) education

Children need to learn to define and identify emotions, developing an appropriate emotional vocabulary (Figure 7.1). They can then learn to distinguish between thoughts and feelings, and to link thoughts, feelings, and behaviour. In a group setting, children can help each other to develop a dictionary of emotions using pictures and games. They can become competent in self rating of emotions, using techniques such as the "feelings thermometer" to rate intensity of anxiety or depression (Figure 7.2). Self monitoring of behaviour can also be developed by recognising and labelling targeted behaviours. Thoughts can be monitored using techniques such as "The Thought Detective" and thought bubbles to identify thoughts in different situations. For older children, training in managing a thought diary can be developed.

An important aspect of emotional education in a group setting is that the group leaders can constantly model expression of feelings and appropriate empathising with others.

Emotional education in groups can also include social skills exercises such as learning to give feedback to others or rehearsing how to give and receive compliments. Other exercises can be added such as identifying positive and negative qualities in oneself, or using pictures, vignettes, or role play to identify what others are feeling in order to promote empathy.

Problem solving

The core elements of problem solving are as follows.

- Define the problem.
- Generate alternative solutions.
- Assess the pros and cons of each solution.
- Decide on a plan to tackle the problem.
- Carry out the plan and monitor it.

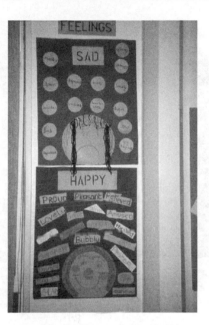

Figure 7.1 Developing an emotional vocabulary

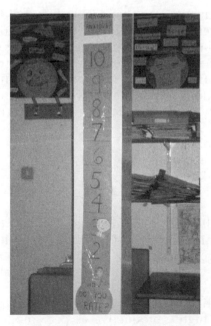

Figure 7.2 Feelings thermometer

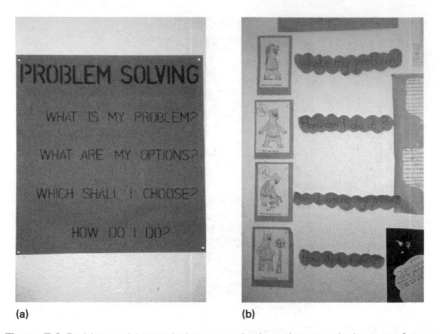

(a)   (b)

Figure 7.3 Problem solving techniques need adaptation to suit the age of group members

These core elements can be adapted for different age groups (Figure 7.3). In very young children, the generation of alternatives before moving on to assess the advantages and disadvantages of each may be too difficult and cause confusion. For children of junior school age, the "Think Aloud" programme[2] teaches children to ask four simple questions when they have a problem, with the aid of Ralph the Bear who asks the following questions (Figure 7.3b).

- What is my problem?
- What can I do about it?
- Is my plan working?
- How did I do?

In generating alternative solutions, an element of fun can be used to loosen rigid thinking by asking what the little green man from Mars might suggest. It is also important to remember that "no change" has to be included as one of the alternatives in the evaluation.

In a group setting, generation of alternatives and evaluation of solutions can be highly productive as peer modelling and ideas of other children will broaden the repertoire of group members.

Children and adolescents who are depressed or anxious and lacking in confidence may need particular help in thinking broadly when generating alternatives. They may also need encouragement to persist with considering possibilities rather than prematurely dismissing a solution before it has been evaluated thoroughly. They can also be helped to consider creative and positive possibilities and then to use these through activity scheduling to increase pleasurable events in their lives.

In contrast, children and adolescents with conduct disorder will often need help to identify their problems appropriately because they are particularly liable to attribute their problems to the hostile intentions of others. They are also likely to need encouragement to consider assertive and non-aggressive alternative solutions to interpersonal difficulties.

Cognitive restructuring

The central aspects of cognitive restructuring include:

- thought identification and monitoring
- linking thoughts, feelings, and behaviour
- challenging and changing distorted and dysfunctional thoughts
- learning alternative ways of coping with difficult situations.

The following paragraphs describe some cognitive restructuring techniques that can be applied in the group setting with children and adolescents.

Children and adolescents in a group can be helped to recognise the dysfunctional negative automatic thoughts that often trigger dysphoric feelings or unhelpful behaviours. Negative automatic thoughts can be identified in a number of ways, such as the use of recall, diaries, role plays, questionnaires or imagery, or by investigating sudden affect changes during the group – "What was going through your mind then? An image? A strong feeling?".

Looking at the evidence for and against a belief and assessing its usefulness provides an excellent exercise for a group. The following questions can be used as prompts.

- What is the evidence in favour of the belief?
- What is the evidence against it?
- Are there alternative ways of viewing the situation?
- What is the effect of thinking this way?
- What would be the effect of changing this way of thinking?
- What are the thinking errors (unhelpful thought patterns)?
- What would you tell a close friend who had a similar belief/ predicament?

83

- What would your friend tell you?
- What can you do? (behavioural experiments/action plans)

Guided discovery and downward arrow techniques can be used in the group setting to elicit meaning – "If this thought were true what would it mean to you?".

Recurrent themes can be identified over time, and activating events or triggers can be reframed as an opportunity to practise coping skills ("show that I can" [STIC] tasks). Groups can also provide the opportunity to carry out instant behavioural experiments such as doing a survey of how much other people notice about you in a social situation, in order to test the thought that everyone is looking at you and noticing you shaking. A group can also be useful to generate positive self statements and positive alternative thoughts contributed by other group members for someone who is depressed.

For young children, thought bubbles and cartoons can be used as a way to elicit thoughts and images, whereas older children can manage a simple thought diary or log.

It is important at all ages that the child understand that it is only their thought that is being challenged. They should not see themselves as being told that they are "wrong" or are being told off.

Therapist characteristics

The style of the therapist is active, positive, and collaborative, without having all the answers. The group should be made attractive and enjoyable for the children, and group leaders need to commit themselves to time outside the group for thorough preparation, debriefing, and supervision. Therapists need to develop a repertoire of therapeutic exercises for appropriate stages in the group, but also need the flexibility and ability to respond to therapeutic opportunities occurring spontaneously.

Overall therapists should aim to "teach in a playful way and play in a way that teaches".[1] They should be able to manage the group so that disruptive behaviour is contained and therapy can proceed.

Techniques and materials

The ethos of the group should be that problems can be solved and the group is an opportunity to learn skills to do this. Group activities form the matrix within which the work of therapeutic change occurs.

Therapists need to have a range of therapeutic materials available, some of which may be home produced or specifically tailored for a

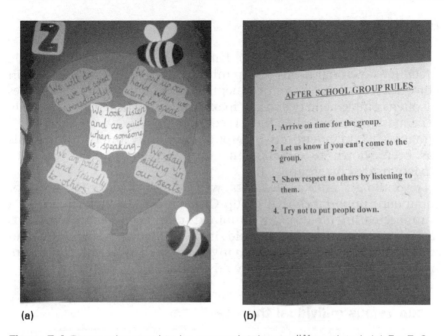

(a)   (b)

Figure 7.4 Group rules need to be appropriately age differentiated. (a) For 7–9 year olds. (b) For 13–15 year olds

particular group, whereas others may be adapted from the range of available manuals (see list below). Video exercises can be particularly useful for those children who find it difficult to empathise with others.

Labelling techniques can help children to develop self talk skills for later use. For example, instead of catastrophising when a crisis occurs, an anxious child can learn to re-label the problem as a challenge and use problem solving to work out the best solution. Activating events and triggers to anxiety or anger can be recognised and managed.

Group rules that are age appropriate can be developed in consultation with the group and may be attractively illustrated in poster form (Figure 7.4).

Useful suggestions for adolescent friendly materials are (Aubin A, personal communication):

- written materials in a file to which the adolescent can always refer
- a web page that is updated after each workshop (for the IT literate group leader)
- use of clip-art packages to liven up handouts
- handouts generated from the adolescents' ideas during groups
- asking for volunteers from the previous group series to help redesign materials for the next group.

The therapeutic framework

Although group CBT has been demonstrated to have a therapeutic effect in its own right, CBT group interventions are usually set within a broad based framework for treatment. Combined treatment approaches are often complementary and can maximise overall benefit. This is likely to be most important when there is co-morbidity.

Many CBT interventions incorporate a family intervention. This has been shown to enhance the improvement of children with anxiety treated by group CBT.[3]

For children and adolescents with conduct disorder it is of paramount importance that group CBT be seen as one element in a multifaceted intervention. A combined multisystem approach needs careful orchestration and should include regular networking and consultation between all agencies involved, such as health, education, and social services, in order to avoid conflict and confusion.[4]

Group versus individual therapy

The group setting is ideally suited to work on social skills with children and adolescents. Groups may make use of overt social skills training as a specific therapeutic intervention but, even without this, groups implicitly expose children and adolescents to interaction with peers. Interpersonal difficulties within the group can be identified and worked on. It is known that social skills deficits are associated with poorer outcome in depression[5] and that, in obsessive–compulsive disorder (OCD), isolation is associated with poorer outcome and the presence of OCD interferes with normal social developmental tasks. Thus, working on social skills deficits in a group is likely to be beneficial.

Within the group process certain aspects have been identified as "curative factors" (also see Chapter 8).[6] These include the realisation that one's difficulties are not unique, and the installation of hope. For adolescents peer modelling and the reduction of stigma are likely to be particularly important. It has also been noted that group psychotherapy tends to have fewer dropouts than individual therapy.[7]

However, it should be noted that, in a recent randomised controlled trial comparing individual CBT, group CBT, and a waiting list control,[8] although both CBT interventions resulted in significant treatment gains compared with waiting list controls, individual CBT was marginally more effective than group CBT. Hypothetical explanations for this finding may include the possibility that, in a homogeneous group in which all group members suffered from anxiety disorders, group members may reinforce each others' fears. Another possibility is that anxious children, particularly those with few social skills deficits, may benefit more from individualised therapy than from the "dilution" that occurs in a group.

Group treatments may offer economical advantages both by enabling up to eight children or adolescents to be treated simultaneously and through the learning opportunity offered to less experienced therapists as a result of working with a more experienced group leader. However, the greater preparation time for a group needs to be taken into account, as does the difficulty of engaging and sustaining in treatment sufficient numbers of group members to maintain the viability of the group.

Homogeneous versus heterogeneous groups

Most research describes homogeneous groups in which children or adolescents with similar diagnoses are treated. For some conditions, it may be an advantage to be grouped with others with a similar problem; for example, in OCD a group experience with other sufferers improves adherence to treatment.

This is not the case for conduct disordered children or adolescents, in whom interaction with conduct disordered peers in treatment groups has been shown potentially to result in iatrogenic effects[9] and may make delinquency worse.[10] Similarly, in a homogeneous group for youths with anxiety disorders (see above), reinforcement of fears between group members may have been responsible for the poorer outcome in group than in individual CBT.[8]

The therapist working with homogeneous groups of children or adolescents with a single diagnosis may experience particular difficulties. Children or adolescents with Asperger's syndrome may change very slowly, and therapists may need support in persisting in work with them. Those working with depressed or anxious children frequently experience a lack of liveliness and spontaneity in the group, which makes the group hard work; those working with antisocial difficulties may experience an "us" and "them" phenomenon, in which the therapist represents a pro-social value system in conflict with the antisocial belief system of the group members. On the other hand, for children with a single diagnosis, working through a specific curriculum can provide a clear supportive framework for the therapeutic intervention. There are now several manuals available for the treatment of specific diagnoses that have been evaluated and found to be effective (see below, under Evidence base and specific applications).

A group CBT programme for a mixed diagnosis group of adolescents with psychological disorders was found to be feasible and to show promising results when used as an adjunct to other treatments.[11] The adolescents had a wide range of psychiatric and developmental disorders. Most had received some type of previous psychological or psychopharmacological intervention but had remaining deficits, particularly in the area of social relating. Each group in this 12 session

Table 7.1 Mixed diagnosis cognitive behaviour therapy group for adolescents		
Session	**Title**	**Treatment focus**
1	Rules for the group, including training between groups	"The story of my problem" (collage)
2	New narrative of skills and strengths	Concept of scaling: worry thermometer
3	Problem solving	Brainstorming, cost–benefit analysis, behavioural experiments
4	Cognitive training 1	Identifying and naming thoughts, feelings, and sensations
5	Cognitive training 2	"Cool thinkers" who think in a more useful way
6	Cognitive training 3	"How I think affects how I feel"
7	Anger coping 1	Awareness of anger; benefits and costs of getting angry
8	Anger coping 2	Arousal regulation using progressive muscle relaxation and guided visualisation
9	Social anxiety management 1	Role play; verbal and non-verbal components of social interactions
10	Social anxiety management 2	Learning how "safety behaviours" make social anxiety worse; role play with and without safety behaviours
11	Relapse prevention	Who will spot signs of relapse? How will they notice? Who can support the young person? Which of the skills learnt will be useful?
12	Graduation party	Group members prepare award for each young person to keep, detailing changes made during the 12 week programme

Adapted from Vickers.[11]

programme lasted for 1.5 hours and started with an activity based on cognitive behavioural principles lasting 45 minutes, followed by refreshments and a short informal social period, and ending with a 30 minute discussion period including lessons learnt during the activity, problems encountered, and solutions. Table 7.1 summarises the content of the 12 sessions. It was concluded that the mixed diagnosis group programme proved a user friendly and clinically valuable adjunct to other treatments, particularly for ameliorating social skills deficits, which, if untreated, may be a risk factor for relapse.

Evidence base and specific applications

The research base for the efficacy and effectiveness of CBT in groups for children and adolescents has been increasing steadily, although it should be noted that there are fewer studies in younger children and that all of the studies cited below are of CBT in homogeneous single diagnosis groups.

Depression

An early school-based group intervention for depression compared the effectiveness of treatment emphasising social skills training through role playing with an approach emphasising cognitive restructuring, both being compared with an attention placebo control and a waiting list control.[12] Children in all four groups showed some improvement, with those in role play improving most followed by the cognitive restructuring group.

The Adolescent Coping With Depression Group Programme (CWD-A) was developed to target the specific areas that are problematic for depressed adolescents, namely discomfort and anxiety, irrational and negative thoughts, poor social skills, and a low rate of pleasant activities.[13] It teaches adolescents to recognise depressogenic patterns of thinking and substitute more constructive cognitions, as well as teaching behavioural skills such as increasing behaviours that elicit positive reinforcement and avoiding negative reinforcement from the environment. This was done through structured group sessions emphasising role playing, homework assignments, rewards and contracts, and incorporating some training in social coping skills. On the assumption that adolescence is a time when many parent–child conflicts arise, leading to mutually punishing transactions, it also included a conflict resolution component.

This programme (i.e. CWD-A) was used alone and also combined with a parent group in a randomised allocation of 59 high school students aged 14–18 and meeting criteria for a diagnosis of depression to one of three conditions: adolescent plus parent groups, adolescent group only; and waiting list controls.[14] Compared with waiting list controls, treated students improved significantly on the depression measures and maintained the gains at two years after treatment. Although there was a strong trend for the results to favour the combined adolescent and parent intervention overall, only one measure achieved statistical significance.[15] Two other randomised clinical trials of the CWD-A programme both demonstrated the effectiveness of group CBT over a waiting list control in adolescents with clinical depression.[16,17]

An adaptation of CWD-A was also found to have a significant preventive effect.[18] Adolescent children of parents with a history of depression who were at risk for, but not yet experiencing, an episode of depression participated in a 15-session after school group package in which they were taught cognitive techniques for identifying and challenging unhelpful thinking that might increase depressive feelings. Compared with a usual care control group, rates of subsequent depression were lower in the treated group, indicating a preventive effect. Prevention is not only preferable clinically but also cheaper than treating the depression once it arises.[19,20]

Anxiety disorders

An 18-session group treatment for children aged 8–14 with anxiety disorders was developed based on the manual by Kendall et al.[21] and making use of the "Coping Cat Workbook".[22] The treatment was largely child focused but several parent sessions were included. The first nine group sessions involved the teaching of coping skills, with the remainder involving exposure to anxiety eliciting situations and practice of the skills previously acquired. The main CBT components were as follows: recognition and labelling of somatic reactions and anxious feelings; recognition and modification of anxious self talk; development of a plan to cope with anxious situations; and evaluation of performance and provision of reward. Compared with a waiting list control group, significantly more treated children no longer suffered from an anxiety disorder after treatment, and treatment gains were maintained at a three month follow up.[7] In a different 12-week group adaptation of the same Kendall programme, similar reductions in anxiety and depression with an improved use of coping strategies was found in children with anxiety disorders.[23] Children whose parents also had group treatment showed greater improvement in their emotional well being and use of coping strategies.

In another modification of Kendall's Coping Cat Programme, "Coping Koala", a 10-week group CBT package combined with three family sessions was compared with a waiting list control group. Significant treatment effects were found both at the end of treatment and at two year follow up.[24,25] The inclusion of family sessions was particularly effective for younger children and for girls.[3]

A pilot CBT group programme for social phobia in adolescence has shown positive results.[26] Key programme components included cognitive restructuring to identify and change the cognitive distortions perpetuating the anxiety, and social skills training to address areas of deficit, together with problem solving training to reduce the tendency of socially phobic adolescents to use behavioural avoidance and escape as coping strategies. Full remission of social phobia occurred in four out of five participants in the group reported.

A single case group design, where 17 children who had witnessed a fire were treated in two groups in which the treatment was staggered, revealed that the symptom count in post-traumatic stress disorder dropped only when treatment was started.[27] The treatment was both psychoeducational and cognitive behavioural. At six month follow up 86% were free of post-traumatic stress disorder.

A pilot study of a 14-week group CBT programme for adolescents with OCD based on the treatment protocol "How I ran OCD off my land"[28] demonstrated clinical improvement and patient satisfaction in this group.[29] Adolescents shared information and designed exposure interventions for themselves and others during the sessions. The protocol included psychoeducation, developing a symptom hierarchy, constructive self talk, cognitive restructuring, and cultivating detachment. Exposure and response prevention interventions were planned and begun in the collaborative and troubleshooting atmosphere of the group, in which the interventions could be discussed and refined. At week seven parents and siblings were involved.

Aggression and antisocial behaviour

A successful school based intervention using an anger coping programme showed treated children to have lower rates of drug and alcohol use, and higher levels of social problem solving skills and self esteem relative to untreated control children at three year follow up.[30] The group programme included training and practice in the use of problem solving, recognition of physiological cues of arousal, and practice in the use of self calming talk during provocation situations. However, as suggested above, there may be iatrogenic effects of bringing together children with conduct problems where deviant behaviour by group members may be reinforced by their peers, resulting in worsened behaviour after the intervention.[9]

For children and adolescents with conduct disorder, the most powerful interventions appear to be those involving parent management training (see Chapter 3). A combination of parent and child training has been found to be superior to either component alone or to a control condition.[31] In older children the interventions showing the greatest successes are those that address multiple risk factors in a comprehensive programme such as multisystemic therapy. Group CBT for children or adolescents may be a helpful additional adjunctive therapy but may be better delivered in a mixed diagnosis group.

Parents are likely to benefit from parent management training in order to reinforce and model pro-social behaviour and social problem solving skills. Parents' cognitions may interfere with the interventions and may need to be challenged. Close liaison is frequently necessary with teachers in order to reinforce developing pro-social cognitions, and sometimes to change inappropriate teacher cognitions and behaviour.

It is important that there is *explicit* work to generalise developing pro-social behaviours at home and at school.

Deliberate self harm

A group therapy intervention called "developmental group psychotherapy" was designed for adolescents who harm themselves.[32] It contains elements of problem solving and cognitive behavioural interventions and additional techniques from dialectical behaviour therapy[33] and psychodynamic group psychotherapy. In a randomised trial, the intervention showed promise in leading to a reduction in repetition of deliberate self-harm, although it did not significantly reduce levels of depression or suicidal thinking.[34]

Social skills

Many CBT group programmes incorporate a social skills component. For young children aged 4–8 with early onset conduct problems, the "Dinosaur School Curriculum" has been developed and evaluated.[31] Elements in this programme include relaxation techniques; recognition of emotions and empathy training; social problem solving skills; anger management; friendship skills; communication skills; and coping in the classroom setting. Compared with a control group, children in the programme showed a reduction in aggressive behaviour at home and an improvement in peer social skills, as reported by parents and observed in interactional tasks. These gains persisted at one year follow-up. Greater changes were achieved when the child programme was combined with a parenting group. Interestingly, teachers did not report changes, which may reflect a lack of generalisation in the absence of a multisystemic approach involving schools in the intervention.

Conclusion

Cognitive and cognitive behavioural techniques adapt readily to application in group settings for children and adolescents, and can be incorporated into effective and enjoyable treatment programmes for a range of problems and disorders. CBT group interventions are best applied as part of a multicomponent package of intervention. Some disorders such as conduct disorder are best managed in mixed diagnosis groups, whereas others benefit from a homogeneous group setting. The evidence base for these interventions has increased steadily over recent years.

References

1 Braswell L, Kendall PC. Cognitive-behavioural therapy with youth. In: Dobson KS, ed. *Handbook of cognitive heightened behavioral therapies*. New York: Guilford Press, 2001:246–94.

2   Camp BW, Bash MAS. Think aloud; increasing social and cognitive skills – a problem-solving programme for children. Champaign, Illinois: Research Press, 1985.*
3   Barratt PM, Dadds MM, Rapee RM. Family treatment of childhood anxiety: a controlled trial. *J Consult Clin Psychol* 1996;**64**:333 42.
4   Bailey V. Conduct disorder in young children. In: Graham P, ed. *Cognitive behavioural therapy for children and families*, 2nd edn. Cambridge: Cambridge University Press, 2003.
5   Goodyer IM, Germany E, Gowrusankur J, Altham P. Social influences in the course of anxious and depressive disorders in school-age children. *Br J Psychiatry* 1991;**158**:676–84.
6   Yalom ID. *The theory and practice of group psychotherapy*, 3rd edn. New York: Basic Books, 1985.
7   Toseland RW, Siporin M. When to recommend group treatment: a review of the clinical and research literature. *Int J Group Psychother* 1986;**36**:171–201.
8   Flannery-Schroeder EC, Kendall PC. Group and individual cognitive behavioural treatments for youth with anxiety disorders: a randomised clinical trial. *Cognitive Ther Res* 2000;**24**:251–78.
9   Dishion TJ, McCord J, Poulin F. When interventions harm: peer groups and problem behaviour. *Am Psychol* 1999;**54**:755–64.
10 Mulvey E, Ashton M, Reppucci N. The prevention and treatment of juvenile delinquency. *Clin Psychol Rev* 1993;**13**:133–67.
11 Vickers B. Cognitive behaviour therapy for adolescents with psychological disorders: a group treatment programme. *Clin Child Psychol Psychiatry* 2002;**7**:249–62.
12 Butler L, Miezitis S, Friedman R, Cole E. The effects of two school-based intervention programs on depressive symptoms in preadolescents. *Am Educ Res J* 1980;**17**:111–9.
13 Clarke GN, Lewinsohn PM, Hops H. *Adolescent coping with depression course*. Eugene, OR: Castalia Press, 1990.*
14 Lewinsohn PM, Rohde P, Hops H, Clark G. *Leader's manual for parent groups: adolescent coping with depression*. Eugene, OR: Castalia Press, 1991.*
15 Lewinsohn PM, Clarke GN, Hops H, Andrews J. Cognitive-behavioural treatment for depressed adolescents. *Behav Ther* 1990;**21**:385–407.
16 Lewinsohn PM, Clarke GN, Rohde P, Hops H, Seeley JR. A course in coping: a cognitive-behavioral approach to the treatment of adolescent depression. In: Hibbs, ED, Jensen PS, eds. *Psychosocial treatments for child and adolescent disorders: empirically based strategies for clinical practice*. Washington, DC: American Psychological Association, 1996.
17 Clarke GN, Rohde P, Lewinsohn PM, Hops H, Seeley JR. Cognitive-behavioral treatment of adolescent depression: efficacy of acute group treatment and booster sessions. *J Am Acad Child Adolesc Psychiatry* 1998;**38**:272–9.
18 Clarke GN, Hornbrook M, Lynch F, et al. A randomised trial of group cognitive intervention for treating depression in adolescent offspring of depressed parents. *Arch Gen Psychiatry* 2001;**58**:1127–34.
19 Andrews G, Szabo M, Burns J. Preventing major depression in young people. *Br J Psychiatry* 2002;**181**:460–2.
20 Schochet IM, Dadds MR, Holland D, et al. The efficacy of a universal school-based programme to prevent adolescent depression. *J Clin Child Psychol* 2001;**130**:303–15.
21 Kendall PC, Kane M, Howard B, Siqueland L. *Cognitive-behavioural therapy for anxious children: treatment manual*. Available from the author, Temple University, Department of Psychology, Philadelphia, PA 19122, USA; 1990.*
22 Kendall PC. *Coping Cat Workbook*. Ardmore, PA: Workbook Publishing, 1992.
23 Mendlowitz SL, Manassis K, Bradley S, Scapillato D, Miezitis S, Shaw BF. Cognitive-behavioral group treatments in childhood anxiety disorders: the role of parental involvement. *J Am Acad Child Adolesc Psychiatry* 1999;**38**:1223–9.
24 Dadds MR, Holland DE, Laurens KR, Mullins M, Barrett PM, Spence SH. Early intervention and prevention of anxiety disorders in children: results of a 2 year follow-up. *J Consult Clin Psychol* 1999;**67**:145–50.
25 Dadds MR, Spence SH, Holland DE, Barrett PM, Laureno KR. Prevention and early intervention for anxiety disorders: a controlled trial. *J Consult Clin Psychol* 1997;**65**:627–35.

26 Albano AM, Marten PA, Holt CS, Heimberg RG. Cognitive-behavioral group treatment for social phobia in adolescents. *J Nerv Ment Dis* 1995;**183**:649–56.
27 March J, Jackson L, Murray MC, Schulte A. Cognitive-behavioural psychotherapy for children and adolescents with posttraumatic stress disorder. *J Am Acad Child Adolesc Psychiatry* 1998;**37**:585–93.
28 March J, Mulle K. *OCD in children and adolescents: a cognitive behavioral treatment manual*. New York: Guilford Press, 1998.
29 Thienemann M, Martin J, Cregger B, Thompson HB, Dyer-Friedman J. Manual-driven group, cognitive-behavioural therapy for adolescents with obsessive-compulsive disorder: a pilot study. *J Am Acad Child Adolesc Psychiatry* 2001;**40**: 1254–60.
30 Lochman JE. Cognitive-behavioral intervention with aggressive boys: three-year follow-up and preventive effects. *J Consult Clin Psychol* 1992;**60**:426–34.
31 Webster-Stratton C, Hammond M. RCT treating children with early onset conduct problems: a comparison of child and parent training interventions. *J Consult Clin Psychol* 1997;**65**:93–109.
32 Harrington R. *Manual for developmental group psychotherapy for deliberate self harm*. Available from the author (e-mail: r.c.harrington@man.ac.uk).*
33 Linehan MM. *Cognitive behavioral treatment of borderline personality disorder*. New York: Guilford Press, 1993.
34 Wood A, Trainer G, Rothwell J, Moore A. Randomised trial of group therapy for repeated self-harm in adolescence. *J Am Acad Child Adolesc Psychiatry* 2001;**40**: 1246–53.

Further reading

References marked with an asterisk in the list above and below are manuals that are useful in cognitive behavioural work in children and adolescents.

Braswell L, Kendall PC. Cognitive-behavioral therapy with youth. In: Dobson KS, ed. *Handbook of cognitive heightened behavioral therapies*. New York: Guilford Press, 2001:281.
Clarke G, Lewinsohn P, Hops H. *Leader's manual for adolescent groups: adolescent coping with depression course*. Portland, OR: Kaiser Permanente Center for Health Research, 1990. http://www.kpchr.org/acwd/CWDA_manual.pdf
Dudley CD. Treating depressed children: a therapeutic manual of cognitive behavioural interventions. Oakland, CA: New Harbinger, 1997.*
Feindler EL. Cognitive strategies in anger control: interventions for children and adolescents. In: Kendall PC, ed. *Child and adolescent therapy: cognitive-behavioral procedures*. New York: Guilford Press, 1991:66–97.
Flannery-Schroeder E, Kendall PC. *Cognitive behavioral therapy for anxious children: therapist manual for group treatment*. Ardmore, PA: Workbook Publishing, 1997.
Graham P, ed. *Cognitive behaviour therapy for children and families*, 2nd edn. Cambridge: Cambridge University Press, 2003.
Hinshaw SP, Erhardt D. Attention-deficit hyperactivity disorder. In: Kendall PC, ed. *Child and adolescent therapy: cognitive-behavioral procedures*. New York: Guilford Press, 1991:98–128.
Kahn JS, Kehle TJ, Jenson WR, Clark E. Comparison of cognitive-behavioral, relaxation and self-modeling interventions for depression among middle-school students. *School Psychol Rev* 1990;**19**:196–208.
Kaminer Y, Burleson JA, Blitz C, Rounsaville BJ. Psychotherapies for adolescent substance abusers: a pilot study. *J Nerv Ment Dis* 1998;**186**:684–90.
Kaslow NJ, Thompson MP. Applying the criteria for empirically supported treatments to studies of psychological interventions for child and adolescent depression. *J Clin Child Psychol* 1998;**27**:146–55.

Kellner MH, Bry BH. The effects of anger management groups in a day school for emotionally disturbed adolescents. *Adolescence* 1999;**34**:645–51.

Kendall PC. *The stop and think workbook*. Philadelphia, PA: Temple University, 1988.*

Kendall PC, Panichelli-Mindel SM. Cognitive-behavioral treatments. *J Abnorm Child Psychol* 1995;**23**:107–24.

Kendall PC, Reber M, McLeer S, Epps J, Ronan KR. Cognitive-behavioral treatment of conduct-disordered children. *Cogn Ther Res* 1990;**14**:279–97.

Lochman JE, Whidby J, Fitzgerald D. Cognitive behavioural assessment and treatment with aggressive children. In: Kendall PC, ed. *Child and adolescent therapy: cognitive-behavioral procedures*. New York: Guilford Press, 2000:25–65.

Mesibov GB. Social skills training with verbal autistic adolescents and adults: a program model. *J Autism Dev Disord* 1984;**14**:395–404.

Nelson WM, Finch AJ. *"Keeping your cool": the anger management workbook*. Ardmore, PA: Workbook Publishing, 1996.*

Ollendick TH, King NJ. Empirically supported treatments for children with phobic and anxiety disorders: current status. *J Clin Child Psychol* 1998;**27**:156–67.

Stallard P. *Think good – feel good*. Chichester: John Wiley, 2002.*

Stark KD. *Childhood depression: school-based intervention*. New York: Guilford Press, 1990.*

Stark KD, Kendall PC, McCarthy M, Stafford M, Barron R, Thomeer M. *Taking action: a workbook for overcoming depression*. Ardmore, PA: Workbook Publishing, 1996.*

8: Psychodynamic groups for children and adolescents

HAROLD BEHR

Overview

A psychodynamic group can be used to provide therapy for children with a wide range of psychological problems.

Careful planning of the group and maintaining a climate of safety are keynotes for success.

A well functioning group can help raise self esteem, offer new solutions to interpersonal problems, and help children to cope with trauma.

Introduction

A psychodynamic group can be used as an effective way to provide therapy for children with a wide range of problems. However, groups can be hazardous as well as helpful, and children are often afraid of being humiliated or isolated in a group. Careful planning is the keynote for a successful group. Every detail concerned with the setting up of the group has to be worked out in advance. Children must be selected who are likely to benefit from the group and be of help to one another, and plans must be made to support the family during the child's therapy. Once the group is running, the therapist must work to maintain a climate of safety. Active intervention is needed to ensure that a child does not become isolated or scapegoated. A well functioning group can raise self esteem, offer new solutions to problems, and help children to cope with illness, loss, and trauma.

Indications and contraindications
for group psychotherapy

Groups provide a therapeutic setting in which the child is expected to interact simultaneously with an adult and other children. On the face of it, this suggests the best of both worlds. However, groups make demands that are not felt in individual therapy. They impose an obligation to help others with their problems, to tolerate not always being the focus of attention, and to deal with a host of challenging interpersonal situations.

The following questions should be asked when deciding whether a particular child might benefit from a group.

How well developed is the child's ability to empathise and identify with others?

Children with a poorly developed sense of self, such as those with a psychotic or autistic disorder, are likely to experience disorganising anxiety and become isolated in a psychodynamic group, although they may benefit from a group structured toward their particular needs.

To what extent does the presenting disorder permeate the child's identity?

Children whose sense of self is dominated by a particular psychological disorder, physical illness, disability, or traumatic experience may benefit in the first instance from a group that is homogeneous for that particular condition. For example, a child who has been sexually abused may need the experience of being with other sexually abused children in a group before joining a group of children with a mixed range of problems.

How does the child cope with interpersonal stress?

Hyperactive children and those with a tendency to resort to physical aggression in the face of slight provocation are likely to reproduce such behaviours in a group. Moderate levels of these behavioural disorders can be contained, but with more than one such child in the group the therapist may find it difficult to sustain a reflective culture.

On the other hand, children who deal with interpersonal stress by being excessively emotionally controlled (for example, those with phobic and obsessional disorders, eating disorders, psychosomatic disorders, anxiety states, and depression) are likely to use a psychodynamic group well, provided their initial anxiety about the relative lack of structure can be overcome. Such children tend to rely heavily on intellectualising defences and controlling manoeuvres at first, but they can usually be helped into more relaxed patterns of relating that pave the way for symptom relief and behavioural change.

What is the child's attitude to group therapy?

Independently of diagnostic considerations, a child who is interested in joining a group and shows curiosity about the make up of the group is more likely to benefit than a child who balks at the idea and only succumbs to parental or professional pressure to join the group. It is, however, possible to engage a reluctant child through preparatory individual sessions in which apprehensions can be fully explored.

What are the parents' attitudes to group therapy?

As with other forms of child therapy, group therapy must be actively supported by parents or carers if it is to be effective. Parental reservations typically hinge on the assumption that psychological problems are contagious, fear that the child will be influenced to behave antisocially, or anxiety that family secrets will be disclosed and intrusive enquiries made into family life. Parents who are reluctant to accept the notion that family relationships might have played a part in the genesis of their child's problems are unlikely to allow the child to enter a form of therapy that rests on such a premise.

Developing an overview of the group

Before working out the practical arrangements, several key questions about the group must be asked.

- From which population of children will the members be drawn?
- Will there be a specific focus or theme, and if so what will it be?
- For how long will the group run?
- Who will lead the group?
- How will the sessions be structured?

It is also worth thinking about what other support systems might be needed while the group is running (family therapy, for example) and what liaison will be maintained with professionals and agencies involved with the child. Parents will need regular contact so that therapeutic change can be integrated into the family dynamic. A parallel parents' group is a good forum for this purpose.

Forming the group

Deciding on the population from which the group will be drawn

Potential group members can be thought of in terms of their similarities and differences. What characteristics will the children obviously have in common, and in what respect will they be obviously different from one another?

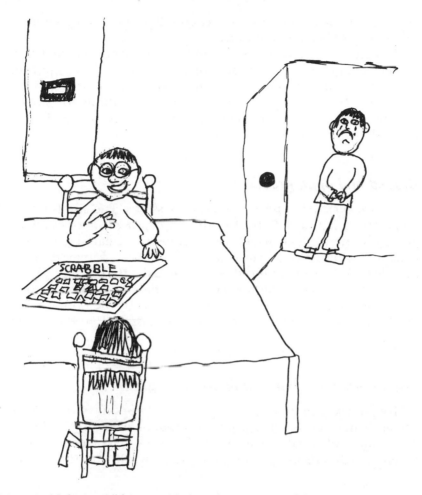

"Not wanted." Some children need help to become part of the peer group

Groups that emphasise similarity can do so in several ways:

- children with similar disorders, for example epilepsy, eating disorder, or post-traumatic stress disorder
- children who have experienced similar life events, for example bereavement, adoption, abuse, or refugee status
- groups for children who share an institutional context, for example hospital ward, residential care unit, or school.

The shared characteristics unite the group in its early stages, rapidly diminishing the child's sense of isolation. Later in the course of the group individual strengths are recognised and different solutions to the same problem are discovered.

Most groups achieve a mix of complementary personality traits and shared characteristics. If possible, articulate and emotionally expressive children should be balanced by inhibited, less verbal children. In practice, however, children undergo surprising metamorphoses in groups, and it is never easy to predict how a particular child will behave in the group.

Closed and open groups

A *closed group* has a fixed number of sessions. The aim is for all the members to start and finish together. An *open group*, or "slow open" group, is one through which the members circulate gradually, each person leaving when a particular goal has been achieved, and new members being introduced to replenish the group. A useful intermediate model allows a group to meet as a closed group for 10–12 sessions, usually on a termly basis, with the option for some children to continue for another block of sessions if further therapy is indicated.

The optimal number of children in a group

Five or six children make up a good working group. Effective therapy can take place in a group with four or even three children, but the element of social challenge and feedback is weakened. Groups of seven or eight are also possible, but are more difficult to contain.

The ages of the children

Groups for children and adolescents tend to fall within several distinct age ranges: 5–7 years, 8–11 years, 12–15 years, and 16–21 years. Within these broad margins, the developmental level and social maturity of the child is more important than actual age in terms of group placement.

Mixed and same sex groups

Each type of group has its advantages and limitations. Mixed groups tend to promote the development of self presentation, whereas same sex groups permit a fuller expression of self doubt and the exploration of more intimate, potentially shameful issues.

Dealing with events outside the group

Dynamic administration refers to the careful attention that must be paid to the numerous events occurring outside the therapeutic setting that have dynamic significance for the therapy and may have to be brought into the therapy. These include messages about absence, communications from parents, carers and professionals, and cooperation with colleagues working in the premises where the group is being held.

Example 1. A mother complained that the therapist was too permissive with her 12 year old daughter, and that the group was inciting her to acts of defiance at home by encouraging her to "stand up for herself". This was dealt with in a parallel session with the mother, but the message also had to be brought into the group, where the child's tendency to play off the group against her mother could be addressed.

Example 2. Several children in a group wanted to visit one of the members, who was in hospital. The therapist discouraged this, framing it positively as a caring impulse but also seeing it as an intrusion into the child's privacy and an infringement of the confidentiality boundary surrounding the group. At an administrative level, the therapist carried the responsibility for conveying the good wishes of the group to the hospitalised child.

Preparing the group room

It is important to secure a quiet and spacious room that will be available for the lifetime of the group. If the therapist prefers to create a setting that pulls children "upward", toward more developmentally mature modes of communicating, then all that is needed is a circle of identical chairs. A more versatile setting involves some play or drawing materials, even for older children and adolescents. Whichever model is chosen should be adhered to throughout the group.

Preparing the child for a group

Group therapy is best discussed first in a family interview. Afterward individual sessions with the child may be needed to prepare the child more for the group, especially if the child has had a bad experience of group life in school.

To allay the fears it is important to describe the group in some detail, informing the child of the ages and sexes of the other children, and even sketching out a few of the problems that they have brought. This "trailer" to the group reduces anxiety about encountering extreme levels of disturbance. Parents are relieved to see that care is being taken in putting together a group of children who are likely to help one another.

To many children, therapy means being made to talk only about the painful and problematic areas of their lives. It helps to tell the child that this is not the case, and that there is no expectation to talk about anything until the child feels ready to do so. The idea of helping other children often appeals, and it enables some children to retain a sense of control in what is potentially an overwhelming situation. The confidential nature of the group is underlined, as are the facts that social contact outside the group is discouraged and that no physically aggressive behaviour is allowed. This generally reassures parents and children alike (Box 8.1).

Box 8.1 Preparing for the group

Describe the group to the family and explain its rationale.
Prepare the child for the group with one or more individual sessions.
Offer parallel therapy to the parents (preferably as a group).
Select children with a capacity for empathy and cooperative play (or talk).
Do not introduce more than one hyperactive child into the group.
Groups for children with a specific shared problem benefit if one of the co-therapists has specialised knowledge of that problem.
Allocate time at the outset for post-group discussion or supervision.

Therapeutic factors in group therapy

The main therapeutic factors in group therapy are summarised in Box 8.2.

Box 8.2 Therapeutic factors in group therapy

The discovery that one is not alone
The group as a place to tell one's story, as a social laboratory, as a mirror, and as a container
Interpretation
The group as a transitional space
The altruistic factor.

The discovery that one is not alone

Probably the single most therapeutic element in a group is the discovery that one is not alone in one's plight. This discovery leads to others: that there is more than one way of coping with a problem; that one can have difficulty in a certain area of one's life and yet have the strength and skill to be of help to others; and that professionals are not the only source of useful information and psychological support.

The group as a place to tell one's story

For many children, the act of telling one's story is therapeutic in itself. Groups have a powerful way of casting light on the shadows of the past. Children who have been harbouring memories of sad, painful, or traumatic events may find, perhaps for the first time, that these memories can be put into words or expressed in play, in the presence of others who are trying to make sense of them. Children are good at supplying one another with words and trading experiences. The therapist is there to ask the right questions, to make links that underline the shared nature of the experience, and to model respectful attention to what is being said.

The group as a social laboratory

In a group it is possible to experiment with newly learned interpersonal skills. Self defeating patterns of behaviour (for example, tendencies to monopolise, disrupt, control others, resort to aggressive or placating manoeuvres, seek an intense attachment to one person, and withdraw from collaborative interaction) tend to be extinguished when spoken about understandingly. New possibilities of relating in a social context are offered implicitly through the availability of alternative models presented by the other children and explicitly through therapeutic conversations.

The group as a mirror

A group enables the child to see himself or herself in others. This can be affirming, but it can also be anxiety provoking, such as when a child recognises his own unwanted traits in others and sets about attacking them. Interventions by the therapist help the child to recognise his own attributes and accept others for who they are. The collective response of the group toward a child also functions like a mirror, reflecting back to the child an image of himself or herself that is less distorted than one which might have arisen in the family context.

The group as a container

Containment is achieved through a balance of acceptance and limit setting. The stability and predictability of the group reduce anxiety. Children for whom excessive control is a problem discover that they can afford to relax and express their thoughts and feelings more adventurously. Children in whom control is too easily lost find that the combined firmness of the therapist and the collective reactions of the group as a whole provide a powerful incentive to regain control and develop alternative coping mechanisms. The group boundary, protected by the therapist from the frequent assaults to which it is subjected in children's groups, reinforces the experience of containment.

Interpretation

Interpretation is a way of linking apparently unconnected phenomena in order to bring about a greater awareness of the origins of a particular problem. The therapist interprets, but so too do the children, to one another. An effective interpretation, couched tentatively and unobtrusively, produces an immediate sense of relief at being understood.

The group as a transitional space

A group reduces the intensity of interactions that are driven by high levels of anxiety, such as hyperactive behaviour, anxious attachment, phobic avoidance, and impulsive aggression. The combination of a consistent structure and an external space creates a climate within which it is possible for children to find new, imaginative ways of expressing themselves. Playful interactions, discussion of dreams, and pictorial self representation all help the child to develop a more reflective way of experiencing himself or herself in relation to others.

The altruistic factor

Expression of the innate urge to be there for other people, even in adversity, is perhaps what makes a group unique as a therapeutic medium. The children in a group know that they are expected to help one another as well as themselves, and this confers on them a sense of importance, duty, and skill that is not evoked in other therapies. The self esteem of the children is boosted by the discovery that they are capable of supporting and advising others despite their own predicament, and that the solutions they have developed to their own problems are copied and appreciated by the other children.

The technique of leading a group

The start of the group

The first group session imprints itself strongly on the children and sets the tone for the rest of the group. The therapist should be active from the outset, leading the process and taking responsibility for determining where the focus of attention should be. A withholding stance heightens anxiety, and one cannot rely on the spontaneity of the children to knit themselves together as a group.

Silences should not be allowed to develop. The therapist can facilitate exchanges by means of open ended questions to individual children, such as "How have you been since we last met?". This prompts personal stories, and opens the way for other children to come in with their own questions and comments. If this does not happen then the therapist can draw them in. Going round in turn is a useful technique for helping each child to find his or her voice. Observations about the group as a whole are generally unproductive except toward the end of the session, by way of a question, for example "How do you all feel now that the session is ending?".

The therapist engages readily in conversation. Later, when the children are confident enough to sustain the interaction themselves, the therapist can afford to be more contemplative, but never for long.

The established group

It is not easy to discern a progression from "superficial" to "deep" as time goes by. Important personal issues can be broached in the first session, and powerful therapeutic shifts can occur at any time in the life of the group. By the same token, a group can become superficial or stuck at any time. Ultimately, it is up to the therapist to judge when the group needs to be steered toward issues that are being evaded.

That said, an established group has a momentum of its own. Children understand that they are there to talk personally, and they report eagerly on the vicissitudes of their daily lives. They exchange information about their families, school experiences, and leisure time pursuits. They offer solace and advice, and kernels of childish wisdom and insight. The therapist should be prepared to engage with any child who seems to be becoming distressed or isolated, or whose behaviour is threatening to disturb the therapeutic culture.

Ending a group

In a slow open group, holiday breaks provide the opportunity for the children to think about their feelings of attachment and dependency and to rehearse the ultimate ending of their therapy. At the start of the group it is a good idea to give each child a timetable containing the dates on which the group is due to meet, and when the breaks will be.

If the group has been a good experience, then the prospect of ending is appropriately tinged with sadness. Children need help to separate from one another by thoughtful discussion well in advance of the ending. It is important for them to talk about whom and what they will miss, what they might have gained from the experience, and how the group could have been better. Sometimes, the prospect of ending brings out earlier anxieties, and the therapist may be dismayed to see some children becoming more demanding at the last minute and slipping back into more immature ways of self expression, but generally these are short lived and give way to mature farewells.

Therapeutic pitfalls

Certain critical moments in groups have the potential to be turned to therapeutic advantage or to develop into bad experiences that set back progress.

The emergence of distressing life events

A group is replete with stories of distressing life events that have a bearing on the very problems that bring the children into therapy. Children talk with candour of family breakdown, abuse, physical or mental illness, and premature or traumatic deaths. Feelings of shame, guilt, fear, sadness, and anger surround these histories.

When a child begins to tell such a story, the others relate what they hear to their own inner world, privately trying to match it with their own experience. Some may offer supportive comments or share their own stories, whereas others may try to distance themselves and resort to diversionary tactics. The therapist has to be particularly active at this point, facilitating the process with empathic listening, questioning, and commenting, but also recognising the need for maintaining protective barriers until a greater sense of safety can be achieved.

Conflict in the group

Children become acutely aware of their differences as well as their similarities. One child may see in another traits that provoke dislike or disapproval, perhaps mirroring his or her own concealed traits. This can express itself in overt criticism and in any of the repertoire of aggressive behaviours learned in the playground, such as teasing, mimicking, accusing, challenging, refusing to cooperate, or even physically attacking.

The therapist must intervene quickly to curtail any of this. It is best to engage first with the initiator, and work with this child until a calmer frame of mind is reached. It is not helpful to allow an argument or conflict to escalate. This can result in one or more of the protagonists dropping out of the group. A group cannot be trusted to police itself either. That is the lonely task of the therapist. Once a more reflective mode has been achieved, the group can be asked to think about the source of the conflict.

Scapegoating

Scapegoating, the ancient human tendency to appoint a creature or person to carry the badness on behalf of the group, sometimes affects therapeutic groups. Children whose view of the world is already resentful and persecuted, and whose solutions to life's problems involve blaming others are more likely to cast a vulnerable group member in the role of the scapegoat. This applies particularly to children who come from a background of deprivation and abuse, and whose self esteem is precarious and rests on the disparagement of others.

Scapegoating can be insidious or it can flare up and run its course in moments, before the bewildered therapist can intervene. It takes many forms, such as persistently ignoring someone, labelling them as ill or alien ("not one of us"), or attributing dangerous or malign intentions to them. To stop the process the therapist must align himself or herself with the scapegoat. They must confront the ringleader of the scapegoating process and confront the group with their projections onto the scapegoat. The therapist focuses on similarities between the scapegoat and the others. Eventually, the therapist helps the scapegoat to look at their own contribution to the process. If scapegoating prevails and the child drops out, there may be a feeling of relief, but the template remains and the cycle is likely to recur unless confronted (Box 8.3).

Box 8.3 Some therapeutic strategies

Divide the time clearly between activity and discussion periods.
Do not allow silences to build up.
Engage actively in the conversation.
Address individual children rather than the group as a whole.
Step in quickly to pre-empt conflict or scapegoating.
Draw in isolated children.
Draw attention to the children's strengths and positive changes.

Age specific modes of group communication

Teasing

Teasing is an ambiguous communication that treads a fine line between affection and aggression. It has a useful social function, teaching children the art of playful give and take, and helping those on the edge of the group to conform to the group mores. Often, however, teasing assumes a sadistic quality and takes the form of scapegoating and bullying. The effect may be to drive a sensitive child out of the group. As with scapegoating, intervention must be prompt, first interrupting it and then helping the group to think about its meaning.

Example. A 13 year old boy arrived in the group smelling of aftershave lotion. This prompted another boy to call him "Pongo", which the other children echoed with hilarity. Another child ridiculed the boy as effeminate. The therapist stepped in, asking the leader of the attack to tell about his own personal experiences of being called names. The therapist then invited others to do the same. This led to a group discussion of teasing and being teased in their families, in which all participated.

Joking

Joking, like teasing, is a useful social device. Groups are frequently assailed by joke telling and wise cracks that can be turned to therapeutic advantage. Jokes provide an opportunity to open up taboo topics such as illness, disability, sexuality, and ethnicity. The therapist has to be quick to challenge jokes that act as a vehicle for prejudice. As with teasing, the therapist has to explore the joker's hidden assumptions and spread the exercise to the group as a whole.

In-talk

The language of children and adolescents is peppered with expletives, repetitive "fillers", and everyday words given a radically different meaning in the adolescent demi-monde. Slang serves to protect the group culture from outside incursions. The element of secret understanding confers power by keeping out uncomprehending adults. When such expressions come to the surface in adolescent therapy groups, the therapist should ask for translations. This serves as a way of looking at differences between the therapist and the group, and relates to issues of inclusion and exclusion.

The specific nature of adolescent groups

Adolescence is an age of extreme attitudes and posturing. The adolescent mentality is particularly prone to idealisation and devaluation, which becomes more pronounced when there is marked stress. This is reflected in strong identifications with "good" or "bad" subcultures, popular heroes or antiheroes, and a set of values that often stand in opposition to the prevailing establishment culture.

These positions are replicated in adolescent therapy groups, where the therapist has to contend constantly with an array of extreme happenings, many of which occur at the group boundary or even right outside the group. Intrusions into group members' physical and psychological space, and disruptive or distracting actions inside and outside the group room are some of the ways in which the therapist's authority and *bona fides* can be challenged.

The guiding philosophy is to put an immediate stop to the disturbing event and steer the process toward the owning of responsibility for one's actions and a search for the origins and meaning of the event. The therapist moves deftly between confrontation and support, constantly amplifying the voices of those youngsters who are trying to reach a more self reflective mode of thought.

Co-therapy and training in a multidisciplinary setting

A group can be effectively led by one person. However, there are advantages to having two people lead the group, especially if the group is focused on a particular disorder or disability, when it helps to have one therapist with specialised knowledge of the condition (a paediatrician or health visitor, for example) working alongside another who has the training to keep an eye on the psychodynamic aspects of the group. In certain groups the sex of the group leaders can be an issue. For example, a group of girls who have been sexually abused by men should have at least one woman therapist.

A further advantage of co-therapy is that it offers a model to the children of how two adults can cooperate. When differences or disagreements arise between the therapists, the group can witness these and join in the attempt to resolve them. This provides a corrective emotional experience for those children who associate disagreement with escalation into conflict, violence, or family dislocation. Children also like hearing their issues discussed thoughtfully by two adults.

Sometimes training considerations come into play, such as the need to provide a learning experience for a student or a training opportunity for a staff member. Trainee co-therapists should not be silent observers. A more relaxed atmosphere is achieved if they enter freely into the interaction, and an inexperienced trainee can often contribute a fresh perspective. Time set aside for regular discussion and supervision of the group is an intrinsic part of the process.

Recommended reading

Dwivedi KN, ed. *Group work with children and adolescents*. London: Jessica Kingsley, 1993.

Evans J. *Active analytic group therapy for adolescents*. London: Jessica Kingsley, 1998.

Thompson S. *The group context*. London: Jessica Kingsley, 1999.

Wright S. Group work. In: Lask B, Bryant-Waugh R, eds. *Anorexia nervosa and related eating disorders in childhood and adolescence*, 2nd edn. Hove, East Sussex: Psychology Press Ltd., 2000:307–322.

9: Family work and family therapy in child mental health

DAVID GOLDBERG, MATTHEW HODES

Overview

Management of child mental health problems may involve contact with parents and families to obtain information, to support the child, to work directly on improving the child's adjustment, or to administer a "prescribed" treatment.

Approaches in family therapy vary as to whether they focus on family interactions, beliefs, intergenerational processes, or narratives.

Family therapy practice has become more eclectic, and frequently used techniques include reframing, use of the genogram, and questioning to change perceptions of relationships.

There is a strong evidence base for family therapy for oppositional defiant disorder and conduct problems, substance misuse, anorexia nervosa, and schizophrenia.

It may also be useful together with individual psychological therapy and psychopharmacology.

Family therapy is versatile because it may be used with families from diverse cultural backgrounds and with a range of structures.

Introduction

Talking with families is an essential part of providing child psychiatric treatments. Children are brought for help by their parents or carers, who are important informants and are usually legally responsible for the child's welfare. Parents and other family members are often involved in implementing interventions to help the child. Even when children and adolescents are seen without a high level of parental involvement, the young person's mental health needs to be seen within the context of their family life, and the child or adolescent is likely to need their family's help at some stage in the treatment process.

This chapter describes many aspects of working with families in child mental health settings. It begins by defining the terms used, making a distinction between generic work with families and family therapy. Because working with families has been strongly influenced by developments in family therapy, different models of family therapy and some of its important concepts are described. The chapter ends with a summary of the effectiveness of family therapy based interventions and indications for family therapy.

Basic terms

"Think family"

This slogan encourages consideration of family issues whenever children present, whatever their problem. A child may want his father to read a bedtime story every night. This may have to occur late if the father is working longer hours. The child may wait for the father to return but this may create tension with his mother, who may not be favoured by the child for the story reading. Thus, a helpful conversation may link family bedtime rituals with parental sharing of child care tasks and the need to take into account the child's feelings toward the parents.

Talking to individuals about their family

Whether children present alone or with a family member, discussion of the family relationships is likely to be relevant. The problem, and how the child responds to it, is likely to affect members of the family. How family members respond to the child may affect the psychiatric symptoms or disorder and how it is managed. For example, the degree of parental consistency, warmth, or hostility to a child may influence the level of disruptive behaviour shown by the child.

Family work

The concept of "family work" refers to therapeutic meetings with family members. The initial task of the therapist is to share information and negotiate the goals of treatment. This proceeds by discussing the situation faced by the family and progressively involving those family members who may be able to help the child and his or her carers. Close family friends, whom the child and parents feel can help the situation, together with the professionals worried for the child's health, can be enrolled in the process.

Family therapy

"Family therapy" is the name given to the therapeutic modality or style of intervention in which the family or network of significant social relationships is seen as the context for change. It is based on the idea that changing family relationships, beliefs, or affect may reduce maladaptive and troubling symptoms or behaviour.[1]

Family therapy focuses on the "here and now". It is often carried out with a team to facilitate reflection on family relationships and beliefs as they emerge in the sessions. A frequently used adjunct is video recording or one way screen for team viewing in order to facilitate review by the therapist, training, and feedback to the family.

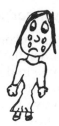

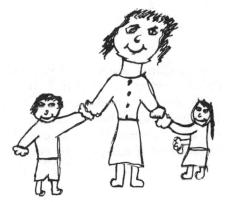

What it feels like to be left out (11 year old). Family therapy can improve the general satisfaction of family members with their life together.

Schools of family therapy and models of change

Family therapy has developed in the UK over the past 40 years.[2] It started with discrete schools of therapy, each of which had a specific model of change, but the number of techniques has increased. The practice of family therapy has increasingly involved integration of approaches. Other frameworks have had a major influence, the most influential recently being post-modern approaches to psychotherapy and psychology,[3] attachment theory,[4] and developmental psychopathology.[5]

Schools of family therapy commonly referred to include the following:

- psychoeducation
- behavioural family therapy
- structural family therapy
- strategic family therapy
- systemic or Milan style therapy
- brief or solution focused therapy
- intergenerational family therapy
- narrative therapy.

Psychoeducation

This involves informing family members about the psychological disorder, the best treatments, and how they work.[6] Family attitudes may change in the light of new information and subsequent discussions. As a specific component of management involving families, this can be effective in discrete child mental health disorders such as first onset psychosis or pervasive developmental disorder.

Behavioural family therapy

Behavioural family therapy applies learning theory to the family context.[7] Modification of the child's behaviour can occur, with the family members acting as co-therapists. In the example of infant sleep difficulties, the parents would monitor their child's behavioural pattern, change contingent factors, and monitor the outcome. For instance, the time of settling or the bedtime rituals may be changed or factors introduced to reinforce the child's return to bed.

Structural family therapy

This is based on the concept of family organisation or structure. The family structure at the time of the child's presentation is thought to be related to the perpetuation of the problem.[8] Changing the family's structure would allow family members to act differently, thus changing the context of the problem.[9] In a simplified example of a child showing tantrums, a structural intervention would ensure that parents respond consistently, and with confidence, rather than perhaps alternating in chastising and comforting him, because this may reflect the child's alternating alliance and their own undeclared conflict.

Strategic family therapy

Strategic family therapy views the child's problem as having a function in maintaining or resolving the family's interactional difficulties.[10,11] The attempt to give up the symptom is seen as perpetuating the problem. Alternatives to giving up the problem are considered, or the problem might even be "prescribed". In order to do this, the symptom or problem has to be reframed (see below). For example, the child who has tantrums might be asked to have tantrums reliably and punctually, and the effect of this undesirable behaviour becoming more predictable and controlled by the parent may then change the interaction so that the tantrums become less frequent.

Systemic or Milan-style therapy

This focuses on the beliefs of family members and how these reflect family organisation. The symptom or how it is understood by each family member becomes part of a network of interacting relations.[12,13] In the example of the child with tantrums, the parents and other family members would be asked a series of questions, the answers to which would elaborate how the symptom influences the pattern of relationships over time. For instance, "How does the child's tantrums affect the relationship between you and your mother?".

Brief or solution focused therapy

This therapy focuses on current opportunities for change while limiting the constraints of the past. For instance, in the stylised example introduced above, questioning could focus on expanding the current strategies that are working (for instance, asking about situations when the tantrums are avoided). Promoting a positive response is encouraged by the "miracle question" – "When you wake up and the problem has gone away, what would be the first thing you notice as different?"[14]

Intergenerational family therapy

Intergenerational family therapy examines how beliefs and patterns of behaviour interconnect across generations. In the example used, the discussion could include similarities and differences between grandparents' and parents' life stories.[15] For example, if a parent has an explosive temper, then it may be harder to feel calm about dealing with the child's tantrums. Understanding these intergenerational processes may be linked to the application of attachment theory.[16]

Narrative therapy

This encourages each person to tell their understanding of the problem they face in terms of stories.[3] During therapy, these narratives evolve as they are interconnected with other persons' stories. A narrative approach would encourage the participants in our example to elaborate their accounts or "stories" of their situation and future.[17] The telling and retelling of stories enables children and their families to think about their problems differently, and this may result in changed behaviour. Depressed children may feel that they have no choices in their lives or that their future is relentlessly pessimistic. Externalisation is a technique to make the problem more manageable by distancing the problem from the child, so that the child can act to manage, defeat, or dissolve the problem.[18]

115

Selected family therapy concepts and interventions

Some important concepts and techniques for intervention are described.

Family life cycle

Everyone in a family will be going through their own life cycle, which can be thought of as a series of stages, each with certain developmental tasks.[19] The child may be progressing from nursery to primary school while adapting to the birth of a brother; the mother may be adapting to having a second child while the father may be increasingly involved in attending to the needs of his elderly parents. Within such a family context, a child presenting with difficulties such as separation anxiety disorder needs to be understood within the context of the family's life cycle demands, which may result in less parental attention and support.

The genogram

Understanding links across generations and family patterns may be achieved by finding out about the family tree, or genogram.[20] Drawing the family tree can involve all family members in discussing relationships and those of the extended family. Considering the presenting issue in the context of the genogram links what is happening for each individual. For instance, a child's separation anxiety may be connected to tasks facing his mother and the support she may need from other members of the family. The genogram places the family's current situation within the context of past life events and changes, such as the experience of the parents in their early schooling. Common themes linking one generation to another emerge, such as parental expectations for their children. These repeating patterns or stories are sometimes referred to as "scripts" if family members feel that they may be destined either to replicate these experiences or to work hard to prevent these events befalling themselves or their children.[15]

Process

Process refers to the sequence or pattern of interactions between people. Observation and discussion of the "here and now" process, which takes place in family sessions, is regarded as relevant to the presenting problem. For instance, discussion of who acts as spokesman for the family or the way in which family members cooperate may connect to the problem or be part of the attempted solution. Discussion of process can lead to clarification of established cycles of behaviour and interaction.[21]

Enactment

Family members can find themselves repeating the same interaction around the problem even if they are trying to change. Enactment is a technique for finding more adaptive patterns of interaction by helping family members to become more aware of the patterns they are repeating. This may be carried out during sessions by the therapist asking family members to "enact" or carry out a discussion of ways of dealing with behaviour in the family (for example, tantrums or defiance in a child), which will help all family members to become aware of their relationships.[9]

Hypotheses and questioning

A hypothesis is a postulated explanation based on available information, such as the referral letter or initial meetings. Working "hypotheses" are used during the meeting with the family. As discussion ensues among family members, and more information is obtained, hypotheses evolve and may be fed back to the family. The term hypothesis is useful because it encourages questioning of assumptions and may suggest new lines for questioning.

Questioning itself can be understood as an intervention with therapeutic potential that can stimulate family members to question their own beliefs, to build up alternative explanations, to give experience of difference patterns of interaction, and to stimulate and plan different ways of interacting. Circular questioning, perhaps the best known style of questioning, requires family members to hear the interconnections between people and their beliefs (what impact one thing makes on something else, usually a relationship).[22] For instance, "What is the effect on your parents of your son going to nursery school?". By asking about differences and how they are connected, new information is generated and shared. "What do you think has changed since your grandmother came to live with you?" may lead onto "What do you think your mother feels has changed since your grandmother came?".

Each family member, and indeed each professional involved, may have different, albeit overlapping, views of the current situation and possible solutions. Exploration of difference – "What has led you to think that?" – may lead to a range of different beliefs and histories. Reflecting on how the situation has arisen might help family members to relate differently.[23]

Positive connotation and reframing

Most beliefs and behaviour, however problematic, can be seen to have positive aspects. Whatever the diagnosis, some aspect of the child's actions can be "positively connoted". A child's temper tantrums may, in a certain light, be seen as showing strength of character, or a girl's anorexia nervosa as having the effect of bringing the family together. The concept of positive connotation can be extended to "reframing". Reframing is an attempt to give a new meaning to a symptom or behaviour, and so widening the conceptual framework. A frequently used example is the reframe of "bad attitude" to that of "growing up difficulties". Such reframing aims to move toward considering undesirable behaviour as a variant of development, and so reduce criticism and aversive interactions.

When children and families come for help they often feel as though there is no clear way forward. Framing this predicament as a "dilemma" may afford family members an increased sense of control. For instance, parents of a drug taking adolescent may feel stuck. By framing their situation as a dilemma, they may be able to think more clearly about the range of ways forward.

Evidence-based practice

An extensive evidence base on the efficacy of family therapy has accumulated, and fuller descriptions are available elsewhere.[24-27] A number of general points have emerged regarding child and adolescent psychiatric disorders.

- Efficacy for family therapy, like all treatments, must be considered in relation to children's age, life cycle stage, and the type of problem or disorder.
- The most effective forms of family therapy are those that include directive elements, specifically behavioural, structural, and strategic therapies.
- Family therapy, or elements of family therapy, may be integrated into other psychological treatments such as behavioural or cognitive therapy.
- Evidence for efficacy of family therapy does not necessarily imply that family relationships and interaction are a cause of the problem or disorder, although family interaction may contribute to the onset, maintenance, or desistance of the disorder.[28]

The following summary of some of the evidence for family therapy is highly selective. Problems and disorders are included if there is at least one randomised controlled trial.

Oppositional defiant disorder and conduct disorder

Behavioural and structurally orientated family therapies lead to improvement for these problems, especially in children, but improvement may also be achieved in adolescence.[29] Increasing consistent parenting, appropriate positive reinforcement for desired behaviour, and reducing coercive interaction between parents and children are among the important components. These interventions share principles with parent management training, which may be carried out with parents and children or modified for groups of parents.[30]

In the USA a more developed variant of structural and systemic therapy, called "multisystemic family therapy", has been used to treat adolescents who show antisocial and delinquent behaviour.[31] This intervention targets the range of factors that may lead to antisocial behaviour, and may include individual treatments, including medication, as well as interventions to address problems outside the family. Although treatment trials suggest that significant benefit can be obtained,[32] a limitation of the intervention is that it is very labour intensive and may not be practical in the UK.

Substance misuse

Many studies conducted in the USA have shown the benefit of family interventions for substance misuse problems.[33] These treatments may have elements in common with family treatments for delinquency and aim to improve family organisation and communication.

Anorexia nervosa

Family treatments lead to substantial benefits for many adolescent sufferers of anorexia nervosa. Family therapy is superior to no treatment,[34] psychodynamic psychotherapy,[35] or supportive psychotherapy.[36] This form of treatment achieves benefit in terms of weight gain as well as eating attitudes and reduced depression, and improves relationships between the parents and adolescent with the disorder, and between the parents.[37]

Schizophrenia

Many studies have demonstrated the benefit of family interventions, especially in families that show high expressed emotion, specifically high criticism and emotional over-involvement with the sufferer. The treatments are an adjunct to pharmacotherapy and psychoeducation.[6,38,39] Treatments aim to improve communication and problem solving, reduce critical comments and over-involvement with the sufferer, and, when appropriate, improve family organisation, influenced by structural family therapy.[40] The research described has been carried out with young adults, including those in their late teens, and it is presumed that the same principles are beneficial to younger sufferers of schizophrenia.

Indications and contraindications

Family therapy and ideas from family therapy are widely used in child mental health in four main areas.

Discrete treatment for a specific disorder or problems

This will be influenced by the available evidence base (described above).

Framework for conceptualising individual symptoms, problems, and relationships

Problems related to coping with life cycle changes (for example, separations or deaths in the family, or leaving home) may be helped by family therapy. Family therapy approaches may also be useful in working with families in which an individual has learning difficulties, when mourning the loss of the ideal child is not achieved and life cycle transitions are hard to negotiate.

Complement to other treatment interventions

There are some interventions that are a mixture of individual psychological treatments, such as cognitive therapy, with techniques used in family therapy, such as externalising.[24] These may be effective treatments for disorders such as obsessive–compulsive disorder.[41,42] Parental and family involvement is also indicated in the management of other childhood anxiety disorders.[24]

Family therapy may also complement pharmacotherapy. In addition to schizophrenia (described above), there are many disorders in childhood and adolescence for which pharmacotherapy is indicated and for which it may be appropriate to provide concurrent family therapy. A good example is the treatment of severe depression, for which family therapy may address specific aspects of relationship difficulties such as critical coercive interactions that are known to perpetuate the disorder.[43,44]

Informing consultations, institutional management, and service developments

Family therapy thinking can be applied to the dynamics of small and large groups, and may be useful in understanding consultation with other professionals, supervision groups, psychotherapy groups, and working in complex systems and organisations such as National Health Service trusts.

Important practical advantages of family therapy are that it can be adapted for use in diverse cultures.[45-47] It can also be used with diverse family forms, including families in which parents are separated or divorced,[48] reconstituted families, and families in which parents are gay or lesbian.[49]

Although there are no contraindications to the use of concepts derived from family therapy, for certain clinical situations and disorders it cannot be the mainstay of treatment. Child abuse or threat of violence is an absolute contraindication, because other agencies and other interventions are typically required. Family therapy is also not indicated as the mainstay of treatment for underlying neurobiological disorders (for example, autism and learning difficulties) and psychoses (although it could be an adjunct, as described above, for helping families to cope better with such problems).

References

1 Gorell Barnes G. Family therapy. In: Rutter M, Taylor E, Hersov L, eds. *Child and adolescent psychiatry. Modern approaches*, 3rd edn. Oxford: Blackwell, 1994.
2 Goldberg D, Jenkins H. Thatcher's family: the development of family therapy in Britain in the 1980's. In: Gielen U, Comunian A, eds. *International approaches to the family and family therapy*. Padua, Italy: CEDAM, 1999.
3 Boston P. Systemic family therapy and the influence of post-modernism. *Adv Psychiatr Treat* 2000;6:450-7.
4 Akister J. Attachment theory and systemic practice: research update. *J Family Ther* 1998;20:353-66.
5 Rutter M. Resilience concepts and findings: implications for family therapy. *J Family Ther* 1999;21:119-44.
6 Fadden G. Research update: psychoeducational family interventions. *J Family Ther* 1998;20:293-309.
7 Crane DR. Introduction to behavioural family therapy for families with young children. *J Family Ther* 1995;17:229-42.
8 Minuchin S. *Families and family therapy*. Cambridge, MA: Harvard University Press, 1974.
9 Minuchin S, Fishman HC. *Family therapy techniques*. Cambridge, MA: Harvard University Press, 1981.
10 Madanes C. *Strategic family therapy*. San Francisco, CA: Jossey-Bass, 1981.
11 Madanes C. Strategic family therapy. In: Gurman A, Kniskern D, eds. *Handbook of family therapy*, Vol 2. New York: Brunner-Mazel, 1991.
12 Jones E. *Family systems therapy: developments in the Milan systemic therapy*. Chichester: Wiley, 1993.

13 Selvini-Palazzoli M, Boscolo L, Cechin G, Prata G. *Paradox and counterparadox.* New York: Jason Aronson, 1978.
14 DeShazer S. *Keys to solutions in brief family therapy.* New York: Norton, 1985.
15 Byng-Hall J. *Rewriting family scripts: improvisation and systems change.* New York: Guilford Press, 1995.
16 Byng-Hall J. Attachment as a base for family and couple therapy. *Child Psychol Psychiatry Rev* 2001;6:31–6.
17 Parry A. A universe of stories. *Family Process* 1991;30:37–54.
18 White M, Epston D. *Narrative means to therapeutic ends.* New York: Norton, 1990.
19 Carter B, McGoldrick M. *The changing family life cycle*, 2nd edn. New York: Gardner Press, 1989.
20 McGoldrick M, Gerson R. *Genograms in family assessment.* New York: Norton, 1985.
21 Cooklin A. Change in "here-and-now" systems vs systems over time. In: Bentovim A, Gorell Barnes G, Cooklin A, eds. *Family therapy. Complementary frameworks of theory and practice.* London: Academic Press, 1987.
22 Selvini-Palazzoli M, Boscolo L, Cechin G, Prata G. Hypothesizing-circularity-neutrality: three guidelines for the conductor of the session. *Family Process* 1980;19:3–12.
23 Vostanis P, Burnham J, Harris Q. Changes in expressed emotion in systemic family therapy. *J Family Ther* 1992;14:15–27.
24 Carr A. Evidence based practice in family therapy and systemic consultation. I: child-focused problems. *J Family Ther* 2000;22:29–60.
25 Cottrell D, Boston P. Practitioner review: the effectiveness of systemic family therapy for children and adolescents. *J Child Psychol Psychiatry* 2002;43:573–86.
26 Diamond G, Siqueland L. Current status of family intervention science. *Child Adolesc Psychiatr Clin North Am* 2001;10:641–61.
27 Fonagy P, Target M, Cottrell D, Phillips J, Kurtz Z. *What works for whom? A critical review of treatments for children and adolescents.* New York: Guilford Press, 2002.
28 Diamond GS, Serrano AC, Dickey M, Sonis WA. Current status of family-based outcome and process research. *J Am Acad Child Adolesc Psychiatry* 1996;35:6–16.
29 Kazdin AE. Parent management training: evidence, outcomes, and issues. *J Am Acad Child Adolesc Psychiatry* 1997;36:1349–56.
30 Webster-Stratton C, Hammond M. Treating children with early onset conduct problems: a comparison of child and parent training interventions. *J Consult Clin Psychol* 1997;65:93–109.
31 Henggeler SW, Schoeenwaald SK, Borduin CM, Rowland MD, Cunningham PB. *Multisystemic treatment of antisocial behavior in children and adolescents.* New York: Guilford Press, 1998.
32 Borduin CM. Multisystemic treatment of criminality and violence in adolescents. *J Am Acad Child Adolesc Psychiatry* 1999;38:242–9.
33 Stanton MD, Shadish WR. Outcome, attrition, and family-couples treatment for drug abuse: a meta-analysis and review of the controlled, comparative studies. *Psychol Bull* 1997;122:170–191.
34 Crisp AH, Norton K, Gowers S, *et al.* A controlled study of the effect of therapies aimed at adolescent and family psychopathology in anorexia nervosa. *Br J Psychiatry* 1991;159:325–33.
35 Robin AL, Siegel PT, Moye AW, Gilroy M, Dennis AB, Sikand A. A controlled comparison of family versus individual therapy for adolescents with anorexia nervosa. *J Am Acad Child Adolesc Psychiatry* 1999;38:1482–9.
36 Russell GFM, Szmukler GI, Dare C, Eisler I. An evaluation of family therapy in anorexia nervosa and bulimia nervosa. *Arch Gen Psychiatry* 1987;44:1047–56.
37 Eisler I, Dare C, Hodes M, Russell G, Dodge E, Le Grange D. Family therapy for adolescent anorexia nervosa: the results of a controlled comparison of two family interventions. *J Child Psychol Psychiatry* 2000;41:727–36.
38 Goldstein M, Miklowitz D. The effectiveness of psychoeducational family therapy in the treatment of schizophrenic disorders. *J Marital Family Ther* 1995;21:361–76.
39 Mari J, Adams C, Steiner D. Family interventions for those with schizophrenia. In: Adams C, DeJesus Mari J, White P, eds. *Schizophrenia module of the Cochrane database of systematic reviews. The Cochrane Library.* Oxford: The Cochrane Collaboration, 1996.

40 Kuipers L, Leff J, Lam D. *Family work for schizophrenia: a practical guide*. London: Gaskell, 1992.
41 March J, Mulle K. *OCD in children and adolescents: a cognitive-behavioural treatment manual*. New York: Guilford, 1994.
42 Waters TL, Barrett PM, March JS. Cognitive-behavioural family treatment of childhood obsessive compulsive disorder: preliminary findings. *Am J Psychother* 2001;**55**:372–87.
43 Asarnow JR, Goldstein MJ, Tompson M, Guthrie D. One-year outcomes of depressive disorders in child psychiatric in-patients: evaluation of the prognostic power of a brief measure of expressed emotion. *J Child Psychol Psychiatry* 1993;**34**:129–37.
44 Kolko DJ, Brent DA, Baugher M, Bridge J, Birmaher B. Cognitive and family therapies for adolescent depression: treatment specificity, mediation, and moderation. *J Consult Clin Psychol* 2000;**68**:603–14.
45 Hodes M. Annotation: culture and family therapy. *J Family Ther* 1989;**11**:117–28.
46 Messent P. Working with Bangladeshi families in the East End of London. *J Family Ther* 1992;**14**:287–304.
47 Wieselberg H. Family therapy and ultra-orthodox Jewish families: a structural approach. *J Family Ther* 1992;**14**:305–29.
48 Kruk E. Promoting co-operative parenting after separation: a therapeutic/interventionist model of family mediation. *J Family Ther* 1993;**15**:235–61.
49 Ussher JM. Family and couples therapy with gay and lesbian clients: acknowledging the forgotten minority. *J Family Ther* 1991;**13**:131–48.

10: Drug treatments

MICHAEL PRENDERGAST

Overview

Psychotropic drugs are generally given by child and adolescent psychiatrists as part of an overall treatment plan, which might include other treatment methods.

Special problems in which drug treatment may be helpful include:

sleep problems

confusion and delirium

schizophrenia

hypomania and bipolar illness

depression

obsessive–compulsive disorder and trichotillomania

tics and Tourette syndrome

anxiety and elimination disorders

hyperactivity

behavioural problems in children with brain disorders such as epilepsy, head injury, and learning disability.

Introduction

Problems with childhood behaviour or emotions that are sufficiently severe or prolonged to interfere with everyday life are classified as psychiatric disorders. Although some physicians distinguish behaviour problems from psychiatric disorders, which they regard as more severe, contemporary child psychiatric practice includes behaviour problems among psychiatric disorders and they are not divided here.

There is general agreement that psychoactive drugs should only be given as part of an overall treatment plan, which will often include other treatment methods described in this book. It might be thought there would also be general agreement that the use of psychoactive drugs should be informed by empirical findings, but there are such large differences in prescribing practices between clinicians and within and between countries that other factors must also be relevant.[1-3] Patterns of use by general practitioners, paediatricians, and child psychiatrists also differ and change. A significant number of

UK child psychiatrists do not prescribe at all.[4] Stimulant drugs are probably the best investigated and best understood psychoactive drugs in use in childhood,[5] and yet they are much less prescribed in the UK[6] than in North America. In the UK, drugs are frequently used to treat childhood sleep problems and nocturnal enuresis,[7,8] which are both conditions that are more appropriately managed with behavioural methods. Thus far, these are unconquered fields for evidence based medicine[9] and often the only supporting evidence available is from case reports and by extrapolation from the adult literature, or from the normal intelligence child literature for children with learning disability.

A number of helpful reviews have recently been published.[10-17]

When drugs are prescribed, prescription patterns follow fashions that the pharmaceutical companies are keen to foster. In national practice, prescription of the latest antidepressant or atypical antipsychotic to children or teenagers should be the exception. Why give new drugs to children with which there is little experience in adults?

Most of the drugs mentioned here are prescribed to children off licence, but this need not be problematic.[18,19] It should be realised that if prescription were limited strictly to evidence based indications and licensed medication, then very few sick children could be medicated at all.

There is still quite a gap between our knowledge of what drugs can do biochemically and why they make some problems better. Most psychoactive drugs affect more than one neurotransmitter system,[20] and so this account leaves neurotransmitters aside and matches operationally defined syndromes with drugs that may improve core symptoms within them. It also tries to place drug treatments within the context of other available approaches.

Drug treatment in the management of specific syndromes

Sleep problems

Difficulty in settling, "midnight intruder", and dawn rising are common sleep problems in the toddler years and respond well to behavioural methods, which are the treatment of choice.[21,22] Prescription of hypnotics to children is contraindicated by the *British National Formulary*[23]; despite this, their use is widespread.[7] Alimemazine (trimeprazine) works well in the short term[24] and may be used in a crisis, for example when parents are severely sleep deprived themselves. Tolerance develops rapidly, and if the response is to increase the dose then the child may become zombie like and drool throughout the day. Data sheets for trimeprazine now contain

125

an expanded section on the risk for tardive dyskinesia, which is another reason for caution. Chloral is an alternative for short term use. Melatonin is discussed below (see under Behaviour problems in children with learning disabilities). Benzodiazepines are best avoided in childhood because they have a toxic effect on behaviour.

Occasional nightmares are common and can follow a frightening experience. If frequent, they should be psychologically investigated. Night terrors, sleep walking, and sleep talking are types of parasomnia and often respond to explanation and reassurance.[25] When they are frequent and occur at a predictable time of the night, they can sometimes be controlled by pre-emptive waking[26]; more usually, this displaces the parasomnia until the small hours. Drug treatment is rarely necessary for parasomnias. Low dose benzodiazepines have been used, and so have imipramine[27] and carbamazepine,[28] which may be preferred.

Narcolepsy and other hypersomnias are seldom diagnosed in childhood. Psychostimulants, for example methylphenidate or dexamfetamine, and more recently modafinil, are favoured in the adult literature. Clomipramine may reduce the frequency of narcoleptic attacks and of cataplexy, which is loss of tone without loss of consciousness.[25] Dietary tyrosine supplements have been found helpful in reducing hypersomnia in adults in some hands[29] but not in others.[30] Quantitative serum tyrosine monitoring is prudent in children.[31]

Confusion and delirium

Confusion and delirium are both medical emergencies and medical assessment is the first line of management. Fever or other signs may point to a medical cause, and non-convulsive status epilepticus is one of many conditions that must be considered. Drugs may be responsible, whether medically prescribed or illicitly obtained, through idiosyncratic reaction or overdose. Enquiries should also be made about traditional medicines and alternative and herbal remedies. When a drug seems responsible for the reaction it should be withdrawn if possible.

Where acute behaviour disturbance is jeopardising treatment, the short term use of haloperidol is recommended,[32] in doses sufficient to confine the child to bed, combined with adequate illumination and sensitive nursing care. Such reactions are usually short lived. Disorientation and behaviour disturbance are often more prominent at night, and chloral is effective if only night sedation is required.

Children with dementing illnesses associated with behavioural problems may rarely require chronic sedation, with chlorpromazine for example, which should be prescribed in the lowest dose effective and at a higher dose at night if night-time sedation is also required. The oral route is preferred because intramuscular injections may be interpreted as attacks. These children's requirements change.

Schizophrenia, hallucinations, and neuroleptic drugs

Schizophrenia of adult type is rare in prepubertal children, although it becomes more common in adolescence. Its management is a specialist matter and will often involve inpatient treatment in a dedicated unit. An underlying physical disorder should always be sought. Treatment is symptomatic.

As drug treatment hinges on neuroleptics (also called antipsychotics or major tranquillisers), with their attendant long term risk for tardive dyskinesia, non-drug alternatives can and perhaps should be tried where appropriate, although it is recognised that most units do not do this. Auditory hallucinations may respond to an ear plug.[33] It should be placed in the more impaired ear where there is a difference, and when the patient will tolerate it. Visual hallucinations are usually paroxysmal, and distorting spectacles interfere with them if the patient can be persuaded to sit down and use them. Both of these types of hallucinations can occur in plain consciousness in the absence of psychosis.[34,35] In these circumstances, compliance with the treatments suggested above may be easier to achieve.

The drug treatment of children and adolescents with schizophrenia is modestly researched, and practice is based upon analogy with the adult literature.[36,37]

It is important to appreciate the huge differences in potency between neuroleptics. A dose of 100 mg chlorpromazine is equivalent to 5 mg trifluoperazine, only 2 mg haloperidol and only 2 mg pimozide, but is equivalent to 200 mg sulpiride and 40 mg clozapine.[15,23] In general, the more potent neuroleptics carry a greater risk for extrapyramidal side effects and the less potent neuroleptics are more sedative, but still have extrapyramidal side effects.

Haloperidol is effective.[38] Inevitably there is far less experience with the new atypical neuroleptics and their long term use.[39–44] They are no more efficacious than the typical antipsychotics and they too are associated with extrapyramidal side effects.

Depending on the degree of disturbance at presentation, sedation may be the first priority. Otherwise, a period of drug free inpatient observation by experienced staff is preferable and may be all that is required in some brief psychotic episodes.

Subsequent management in those requiring medication will comprise a systematic trial of several weeks of a typical or an atypical neuroleptic, given individually according to tolerance. Unfortunately, a therapeutic margin between symptom relief and side effects can be hard to find in the prepubertal patient.[45]

If the response to neither of two neuroleptics is satisfactory after six to eight weeks at recommended doses, then current practice is to move to clozapine quickly. Clozapine offers real hope for treatment resistant patients,[46,47] but in the UK it is only available for use in children older than 12 years subject to compliance with an expensive monitoring procedure to guard against agranulocytosis.

Depot neuroleptics are avoided until a stable response has been obtained, and are better avoided altogether.

Drug treatment mainly affects the positive symptoms of hallucinations and delusions. It has less effect on the motivationless negative symptoms that some patients are left with.[46]

It is not a good idea to make drug adjustments just before discharge from hospital. Once control is achieved, medication should be continued for 12–24 months after recovery.[37] The issue of continued treatment should be kept under continual review. Ciompi[48] has drawn attention to the various patterns of schizophrenic illness. Not all imply "medication for life".

Antiparkinsonian agents are not prescribed routinely but are given only if parkinsonian side effects occur.[49]

Patient and parents must be warned of the possibility of writhing, dystonic movements of the face and body, and oculogyric crisis during the first few days of treatment with neuroleptics, and of parkinsonian symptoms of rigidity, akinesia, tremor, and salivation in the succeeding weeks. All of these symptoms usually respond to antiparkinsonian agents or reduction in medication. Acute dystonic reactions are distressing and constitute medical emergencies. The parents of children who are managed as outpatients may be given a few procyclidine tablets or equivalent to use, if required, pending attendance at a casualty department. Intramuscular injection of an antiparkinsonian drug will bring more immediate relief.

The typical onset intervals for neuroleptic induced extrapyramidal disorders are summarised in Table 10.1. Some patients experience akathisia, an unpleasant restless agitation, usually within the first two months of starting a neuroleptic. It can be difficult to treat without drug reduction. Adult work indicates that akathisia is relatively resistant to antiparkinsonian drugs. Iron deficiency should be

Table 10.1 Typical onset intervals for neuroleptic induced extrapyramidal disorders

Extrapyramidal disorder	Onset interval
Acute dystonias (oculogyric crisis, etc.)	Within hours to seven days
Akathisia	Within hours to three months
Parkinsonism (akinesia/rigidity/tremor)	Within first month
Tardive dyskinesia	Usually after three months
Tardive akathisia	Usually after months
Tardive dystonia	Three days to 11 years
Neuroleptic malignant syndrome	At any time

corrected.[50] Propranolol may be helpful and clonazepam has been used to treat adolescent akathisia.[51]

More seriously, neuroleptic malignant syndrome may present at any time.[52,53] In its florid state it is characterised by fever, fluctuating consciousness, autonomic instability, increased tone, and raised serum creatine kinase. Formes frustes occur and fever or raised enzymes may be lacking. It is a potentially lethal condition. Neuroleptics must be stopped at once. Bromocriptine, dantrolene, and electroconvulsive therapy have been used, but the essence of treatment is attention to fluid balance and cardiorespiratory support in a medical setting. Symptoms may take a week or more to respond but longer if the patient has taken a depot neuroleptic.

Tardive dyskinesia is an important long term risk with neuroleptic treatment. It may be transient and appear as a withdrawal dyskinesia lasting from days to several months or longer,[54] or it may be persistent.[55] In tardive dyskinesia irregular choreoathetoid movements occur predominantly in the buccal–lingual musculature and at the distal extremities. These dyskinesias are not uncommon in children exposed to neuroleptics. Learning disabled patients are at greater risk – 34% in one series[55] – and are also at greater risk for being given neuroleptic treatment. Tardive dystonia is a more malignant variant that is characterised by sustained contraction of skeletal musculature, which manifests as, for example, sustained tongue protrusion, disabling posturing, stridor from laryngospasm, and dysarthria.[10,55–57]

In addition, Gualtieri[10] has described a late onset behavioural equivalent of tardive dyskinesia that he termed "tardive akathisia with dysphoria and restlessness".[57]

All of these conditions are difficult to treat beyond withdrawal of neuroleptics and waiting. If antipsychotic medication is still required, then a switch to clozapine should be considered.[58,59] A minority of patients have *paradoxical* tardive dyskinesia and respond to *increased* anticholinergics.[60] Tetrabenazine may help the others.[61] In contrast to an earlier report by the same group, a later double blind trial of vitamin E showed no benefit in adults.[62]

The unwanted movements may be irreversible but, fortunately, remission rates in children are higher than in adults.[10,13,55]

These are the reasons why this reviewer has tried to avoid neuroleptics. There is a place for them in the management of schizophrenia[37] and Tourette syndrome.[63]

There is never an indication to use more than one neuroleptic at the same time.

Drug holidays are out of fashion and, in the case of neuroleptics, may increase the risk for developing tardive dyskinesia. However, discontinuation, in order to assess the need for continuing treatment and side effects, should be a regular part of the management plan.[57]

Non-extrapyramidal side effects of neuroleptics include weight gain, especially with risperidone,[64] gynaecomastia, galactorrhoea, amenorrhoea, and jaundice. Chlorpromazine is particularly associated with photosensitive reactions and clozapine causes hypersalivation.[65,66]

Thioridazine, droperidol, and sertindole have all been withdrawn recently because of a risk for cardiac arrhythmias from QT interval prolongation.[67]

Hypomania and bipolar illness

Hypomania is characterised by elevated mood, excitement and irritability, pressure of talk, and flight of ideas, which are often grandiose. Teenagers are disinhibited and sleep little. Mania is a more florid version of the same. It is rare before the teenage years. In the acute phase, sedation with a major tranquilliser and hospital admission may be required. Hypomanic episodes may be recurrent, or more usually part of a bipolar illness. Children and teenagers with bipolar disorders have recurrent episodes of severe depression and hypomania.

Lithium carbonate is the treatment of choice.[68-71] Because of differences in bioavailability, it is important to choose a preparation and stay with it. Modified release lithium carbonate can be given once a day and blood concentrations are monitored in the steady state, 12 hours after the previous dose. In practice this means about five days after the last dose increase. Target serum concentrations are usually within the range 0.6–1.0 mmol/l. When control is obtained, measurements are repeated every two months[13,72] and tests of thyroid and renal function are conducted every six months, but more often if there is cause for concern. Fluid loss through vomiting, diarrhoea, and sweating in hot weather can all cause toxicity characterised by diarrhoea, vomiting, tremor, ataxia, dysarthria, and muscular weakness progressing to cardiac arrhythmia, stupor, and death if lithium is continued. Less severe side effects include weight gain, polydipsia, and polyuria. Previous worries about nephrotoxicity appear to have been misplaced.[73-75] Thyroid replacement will be required if hypothyroidism appears; hyperparathyroidism may also occur.[76]

Clozapine may be effective in refractory or rapid cycling bipolar disorder or schizoaffective disorder.[77,78]

Sodium valproate and carbamazepine can be used as an alternative to lithium carbonate in unresponsive patients and may be tried first.[70,79-82] More recently, lamotrigine has been used for the same purpose.[83,84]

In rapid cycling bipolar illnesses, there are three or more occurrences within a year. Sometimes there may be several mood swings within a week or even each day. Thyroid[85] or parathyroid[86] dysfunction may need correction. Sodium valproate or carbamazepine are treatments of choice in rapid cycling patients[87-89] and it may be hard to treat. Dosages are the same as in the treatment of epilepsy, and the sustained release carbamazepine preparation is preferred. Drug levels are not indicated unless there are concerns about compliance.[90]

Carbamazepine may be specific for the periodic psychosis of adolescence described by Yamashita.[91]

Depression

Depression of adult type is increasingly recognised in childhood. In the past it was probably included in the category of emotional disorders without further differentiation.

When depression is suspected, the child must be interviewed alone and suicidal ideas inquired after. A decision should be made whether referral for inpatient treatment is required. Mild to moderate depression responds to cognitive behaviour therapy. Severe depression probably does not.[92] Although child psychiatrists have traditionally used tricyclics to treat successfully the more serious depressions, with depressed mood (as opposed to irritable mood) and melancholic features, evidence from double blind trials to support this practice is lacking. Harrington[93] suggests possible reasons for this discrepancy – perhaps "the use of the rather broad criteria of DSM III has led to the inclusion of a very heterogeneous group of depressive conditions only some of which will respond to tricyclics", particularly among co-morbid study populations, in which depression was diagnosed by questionnaire to obtain subjects from among children attending clinics with some other primary complaint. In the past decade there has been a shift in preference to the serotonergic antidepressants,[1,3] initially because there was no evidence for or against their use in children. Contemporary prescribing is now on a more positive basis for fluoxetine.[94,95] The side effects of these drugs are similar to tricyclics (i.e. anticholinergic, despite their SSRI [selective serotonin reuptake inhibitor] acronym) and include insomnia in the case of fluoxetine. Serotonergics can also cause extrapyramidal disorders.[96-98]

Their peculiar risk is the provocation of serotonergic syndrome, which is characterised by the rapid development of mental state changes, restlessness, shivering, myoclonus, tremor, unsteady gait, brisk reflexes, fever and autonomic changes, including sweatiness. It is usually self limiting if the offending drug is stopped. Active management, if required, is symptomatic in a medical setting. By contrast, neuroleptic malignant syndrome usually develops more slowly (3–9 days). Rigidity, cogwheeling, and catatonia are characteristic, and nearly never present in serotonergic syndrome, and autonomic symptoms are less intense.[99-101] Serotonergic syndrome seems particularly likely to occur when a serotonergic drug is stopped or changed for another.[15]

Antidepressants may cause a manic switch of symptoms in previously unrecognised bipolar patients.[102–104]

Tricyclics still have a place in the management of severe depression that is unresponsive to serotonergic antidepressants.[105,106] Typically, amitriptyline is used for its sedative effect in the agitated patient, and imipramine is used for its more stimulant effect in the patient who has slowed up. Patients and parents should be warned about the early appearance and resolution of the anticholinergic effects of dry mouth, constipation, and blurred vision. These are not usually problematic if the drug is introduced slowly. A baseline electrocardiogram (ECG) is required because a conduction disorder is a contraindication. Children appear to require 75–100 mg/day on average and, starting at 25 mg at night, the dose can be increased by a similar increment every three days or so. Intersubject variation in absorption of imipramine is considerable, and monitoring of blood concentrations is recommended when this tricyclic is used. Puig-Antich et al.[107] suggested that a total plasma concentration of 150 micrograms/l (imipramine and desipramine) is necessary for therapeutic effect. Serial ECG records are recommended if high doses of imipramine are needed to achieve this.[13] The antidepressant effect is not usually obtained before about 10 days of treatment at the appropriate dose.

In treatment responders antidepressants are usually continued for 4–6 months after response is obtained.[108,109] Withdrawal of antidepressants should not be attempted at critical times, for example at the start of the new school year. Parents must understand the need to supervise the taking of tablets and to keep them away from the patient and younger siblings. Childproof containers are essential.[110]

Sleep deprivation or deprivation of rapid eye movement sleep as treatments for depression have yielded inconsistent results but may offer a treatment alternative for antidepressant resistant patients.[111–113]

In seasonal affective disorder, recurrent autumn/winter depression remits in the spring and is often associated with carbohydrate craving, over eating, weight gain, and over sleeping. It responds to light therapy[114,115] started in the autumn or annual antipodal migration. Dawn simulation is an alternative presentation of light treatment for children who will not sit in front of the light box for the required period.[116]

Catatonia has many causes. Affective disorders are the most frequent psychiatric cause. Catatonia will often respond to high dose lorazepam,[117] allowing treatment of the underlying psychiatric or medical illness to be addressed.

Very severe depressive illness that is unresponsive to antidepressants, depressive stupor, and catatonic stupor are rare indications for electroconvulsive treatment. It should not be undertaken without further supportive consultant opinions, perhaps from colleagues in adolescent psychiatry and adult psychiatry, in addition to thorough discussion with patient and parents. The great advantage of electroconvulsive treatment is rapid relief when it is successful.[118]

Obsessive–compulsive disorders and trichotillomania

The manifestations of obsessive–compulsive disorder include repetitive washing, avoiding, counting, checking, and other rituals and compulsions that often involve the whole family. Children who are severely incapacitated by these symptoms may require inpatient treatment.

Behavioural management has a role but it is less powerful in this condition than was originally thought. The serotonergic drugs clomipramine, fluvoxamine, and fluoxetine are effective, even in the absence of coexisting depressive symptomatology,[16,119–121] as is sertraline.[122] In refractory cases clomipramine is usually the third drug tried, if it has not been used already.

Trichotillomania also responds to clomipramine,[173] but this should not be taken as proof that the nature of these two conditions is similar.

Tics and Tourette syndrome

Simple motor tics are widespread, transient, and can usually be managed with explanation and reassurance. The syndrome of Gilles de la Tourette comprises multiple motor tics and phonic tics. Medication is only indicated when the tics are intrusive and handicapping; complete suppression is not the goal as this is seldom achieved. There is no evidence that early treatment modifies the course of the disease.

Haloperidol is best researched and often cited as the treatment of choice.[63] Acute extrapyramidal reactions are common and patients should be warned of the possibility of tremor, stiffness, and oculogyric crisis, all of which will respond to antiparkinsonian agents, for example procyclidine. Antiparkinsonian drugs should only be taken if these problems arise. Haloperidol can cause excessive sedation, which has been termed a "fog" state.[124]

Pimozide,[125] sulpiride,[126] fluphenazine,[127,128] and risperidone[129,130] can also cause extrapyramidal reactions but are less likely to than is haloperidol. Pimozide is less used now because of reports of sudden death due to arrhythmias at high doses. Prior ECG and subsequent monitoring is advisable and a response will usually have been achieved by 8 mg in a single daily dose if it is going to occur.

Clonidine has its advocates and has the advantage that it is not a neuroleptic, but there are doubts about its efficacy[16] and it is said that it may take several months to work. The author finds that it causes depression and does not usually affect the tics at all. Clonidine should not be stopped suddenly but over three or four days in order to decrease the risk of withdrawal symptoms and hypertensive rebound.

Phonic tics are usually the first to respond to drug treatment, and then complex motor tics and then simple motor tics centripetally.

Tourette syndrome may be associated with other psychopathology, particularly obsessive–compulsive symptoms. Rhythmic complex movements that appear compulsive, for example repetitive kissing or lining up, are called complex tics in the American literature, but because they appear to lie between Tourette syndrome and obsessive–compulsive disorder they are perhaps best referred to as "complex movements". Sometimes these complex movements are the main problem. Neuroleptics usually leave them untouched but they will often respond to clomipramine where specific treatment is required.

Tics wax and wane but some children go into "status tic" – a sequence of unrelenting tics and complex movements that leaves them sore and exhausted. In the absence of a more specific remedy, prolonged chloral induced sleep will sometimes bring relief.

Naturally there are concerns about the lifetime risk for tardive dyskinesia in this new cohort of children receiving long term neuroleptics.[131] Treatment alternatives include nicotine transdermal patches (7 mg for 24 hours on a single day each month), which are less invasive and easy to try,[132] and tetrabenazine.[61]

Anxieties, panic attacks, and school refusal

Situational anxieties or phobias are best treated with behavioural methods. In school refusal in the younger child, anxieties are multifactorial and early return to school is the cornerstone of management.

Free floating anxiety and panic attacks may be associated with hyperventilation, which can be assessed in the clinic. Anxiolytics have been used but results conflict as to their efficacy. Serotonergic drugs are probably most popular[3] and there is evidence for the use of fluvoxamine.[133] Benzodiazepines are best avoided because of their addictive potential and propensity to behavioural side effects. Propranolol may be helpful but is contraindicated when there is a history of asthma or arrhythmia. It has the advantage that it can be taken "as required". The tricyclic drugs amitriptyline and imipramine can be given for their anxiolytic effects. The present generation of monoamine oxidise inhibitors is difficult to use because of the food restrictions required to avoid a pressor reaction. The newer reversible inhibitors of monoamine oxidase, moclobemide for example, may make this category of drugs more available to teenage patients, but they too require food restrictions and there are potential problems in switching to other psychotropics.[134]

Hysterical disorders, eating disorders, and chronic pain

Hysterical and somatising disorders are included here because they are sometimes complicated by depression, which should be diagnosed and treated in the usual way. Likewise, depression is sometimes found in chronic fatigue syndromes and anorexia nervosa.

Abreaction with intravenous amylobarbitone[135] can be helpful in the diagnosis of psychogenic stupor and in the management of children with severe non-organic loss of function.[136]

There is no specific drug treatment for anorexia nervosa, but both imipramine and fluoxetine have found support in the treatment of adults with bulimia nervosa.[137]

Gabapentin, carbamazepine, and tricyclics have been used for neuropathic and intractable pain,[138] but in the absence of more specific remedies the management of chronic pain in childhood pivots upon rehabilitation back into normal life, which is regular school attendance. Paediatric rheumatology services often have the best arrangements for doing this and provide useful models.

Elimination

Unlike constipation, the management of encopresis is not usually undertaken before age four years for developmental reasons. Management is mainly behavioural, rewarding stool in toilet. Constipation is frequently associated and laxatives may be required. The choice of laxative is important, but "sister's favourite" is often prescribed by default. The topic has been expertly reviewed by Clayden[139] and is not discussed further here. See also a recent review of constipation in children with disabilities.[140]

Likewise, developmental considerations determine that nocturnal enuresis is not usually treated actively before age five years. Recent onset enuresis may be drug related.[141] There is abundant evidence that behavioural methods are the treatment of choice after physical causes have been rejected. Some children respond to simple star charts rewarding dry nights. Other children require a night trainer alarm that uses the same principle as the bell and pad and is equally effective but more convenient.[142] Many districts now have enuresis clinics to provide this service. Despite the above, amitriptyline and imipramine are still widely prescribed for nocturnal enuresis by general practitioners[7] and child psychiatrists.[8] Although effective in the short term, relapse is frequent when the drug is stopped and the risk for overdose by patient or siblings is well known.[110] There may be a place for prescribing one of these drugs in the short term, for example to allow a child to go on a school holiday, and the same can be said for desmopressin,[143] which is now also available as an oral preparation. Desmopressin may cause headache and loss of appetite, and convulsions, perhaps by water intoxication.[144] With the availability of safer, more effective behavioural methods, chronic drug treatment for nocturnal enuresis cannot be endorsed.

In daytime wetting, behavioural methods including regular potting are the mainstay of treatment, but paediatric urodynamic review should be considered, particularly when there is associated urgency. Most of the drugs used by urodynamicists can provoke nightmares.

Hyperactivity

Children with pervasive short attention span and restless, over active, distractible behaviour meet criteria for hyperkinetic disorder according to the *International Classification of Diseases*, 10th revision[145] and attention deficit/hyperactivity disorder in the American system *Diagnostic and Statistical Manual of Mental Disorders*, IVth edition, text revised.[146] Attention deficit/hyperactivity disorder defines a much broader group because it also includes situational expression of these problems and it is not further discussed.

Hyperkinetic disorder, narrowly defined, is of early onset and occurred at a rate of 17 per 1000 boys aged 6–8 years in the East London study.[147] UK child psychiatrists have been reluctant to make this diagnosis but usually identify the conduct disorder with which it is often associated.[148] It is a disabling condition. Management is difficult and requires attention to structure and consistency, which usually involves environmental manipulation. Stimulant drugs are widely used in the USA[5] but less often in the UK.[6] They are probably the best researched psychotropic drugs in use in childhood. Very many studies have demonstrated their efficacy.[5,149–151] Even though these drugs are reserved for the most severely afflicted children who show this behaviour at home, at school, and in the doctor's office, every health district has candidate patients and each district needs arrangements for these patients.[152]

After diagnosis, baseline parent and teacher ratings (with consent), using the Rutter[153] or Conners[154] scales, are completed, which takes a few minutes. These can be repeated serially to assess change. Methylphenidate[155] and dexamfetamine[5] are both effective. A yes/no effect is sought. When there is a benefit it is clear, and the school dinner lady will notice if a tablet is forgotten. What is more, the child's improved behaviour is likely to have a positive effect on family interaction.[156] If conduct disorder is associated, it will usually be left untouched by stimulants and it is important to recognise the distinct nature of these remaining symptoms and not to expect a drug solution to them. Associated anxiety predicts a poorer response to stimulants.[151,155]

Methylphenidate has a short half life and it is given in divided doses in the range of 0.3–1.5 mg/kg per day, starting with about 5 mg twice a day with a top total daily dose of 60 mg, depending on the size of the child.[5,151] Appetite suppression is sometimes a problem, and so it is usually given after breakfast, after lunch, and possibly after school. Evening doses are likely to cause insomnia.

Reversible growth failure is reported and is probably related to high dose regimens. Nevertheless, height, weight, and blood pressure should be measured at each clinic attendance and this means the clinic should be equipped to do this. Some children become tearful or depressed, and others may develop obsessive–compulsive behaviour[157] or tics.[158] There is disagreement as to whether stimulants should be given to hyperactive children with tics.[13,159] Tics are not a definite contraindication and decisions need to be made on a case by case basis.[16]

Dexamfetamine is longer acting and may be given twice a day. It is usually started at 5 mg/day, with a top total daily dose of 40 mg.[5] The side effects are similar to those of methylphenidate. Some children tolerate one of these drugs more readily than the other. Although both dexamfetamine and methylphenidate are controlled drugs, dependence is not a problem with the doses described here. Sustained release preparations of both dexamfetamine and methylphenidate are now available[5] and may allow a balance to be struck between efficacy and side effects that is impossible with the parent compounds.[160]

If stimulants are effective, then long term treatment and supervision should be anticipated. In the teenage years periodic attempts can be made to reduce and stop them at non-critical times, but it is not necessary to persist with a trial of reduction if there is obvious behavioural deterioration.

Low dose imipramine is a useful but less potent alternative to stimulants[161,162] and is helpful if there is co-morbid anxiety. Carbamazepine is also effective for hyperkinesis and is probably underused.[163]

Clonidine is quite widely used but there is only limited evidence that it is more effective than placebo and its effect is modest.[16,162,164] Guanfacine may be better.[16,165]

Buproprion (amfebutamone) is a further alternative[16,166]; it is contraindicated in seizure disorder. Pemoline has been withdrawn in the UK.

A few hyperactivity specialists are using combination therapy (for example, stimulants and clonidine, or stimulants and risperidone). An increase in their number is not required.

Drug treatments for behavioural problems in children with brain disorders

Behaviour problems in children with epilepsy

Children with epilepsy are at much greater risk for behaviour problems. The reasons for this are multiple but only drug issues are considered here.

It is profitable to review the anticonvulsants the child is taking. If the patient is "known to have epilepsy" then the diagnosis should be reviewed. Surveys of diagnosis in children with epilepsy show that up to 40% have another diagnosis and do *not* have epilepsy.

According to timing, problematic behaviours in children with epilepsy can be described as *pre-ictal*, including the prodrome, or working up to a fit; *ictal*, which includes aura and transient cognitive impairment; *post-ictal*, for example fugue states; and *inter-ictal*, which are the majority, because most people are having fits less of the time than when they are not.

The particular behaviour problems associated with epilepsy are pervasive hyperactivity, depression, confusional states, psychoses, and dementia. All of these can be caused by drugs, and their appearance should prompt review of anticonvulsants and other medication. The evidence for an association between epilepsy and depression in children is not strong as compared with that among adults attending epilepsy clinics, perhaps because the most popular paediatric anticonvulsants are also mood stabilisers.

Pseudoseizures are also more common in those who have epilepsy than in those who do not.

Some anticonvulsants are more likely to cause behaviour problems than others: sodium valproate, carbamazepine, and lamotrigine might do but are less likely to; ethosuximide, topiramate, gabapentin, and phenytoin can do; and clobazam, clonazepam, vigabatrin, and phenobarbital (phenobarbitone) have a high probability. There are early reports for zonisamide. The jury is still out for tiagabine, oxcarbazepine, and levetiracetam. Besag recently provided a useful review.[167]

The behavioural side effects of carbamazepine are often associated with peak serum concentrations. A switch to the retard preparation at the same total daily dose is easy to do and will seldom result in decreased seizure control[168] or deteriorating behaviour, but sometimes produces a gratifying behavioural improvement.

The behavioural side effects of phenobarbital are well known, and paediatricians hardly use it outside the neonatal period, but some adult specialists who also treat children are unfamiliar with this side effect.

Clonazepam and clobazam can both cause profound and chronic behavioural deterioration, even pseudodementia if parents do not decide to stop giving them.[169] Hyperactive children with learning difficulties and intractable seizures who have been on a benzodiazepine from an early age are particularly at risk that drug induced behaviour will be assumed to be constitutional.[170] There is sometimes cross-reactivity between clonazepam and clobazam but sometimes not, and so it is worthwhile to try a switch because benzodiazepine withdrawal needs to be very slow and parents must be prepared for the possibility of seizure exacerbation.

Vigabatrin has made a notable contribution to childhood psychopathology and can produce a spectrum of problems, including psychosis. It is less used now because it can also cause visual field reduction.

Topiramate can cause alarming loss of appetite and weight loss.

One is reluctant to treat *anticonvulsant induced* hyperactivity with stimulants. Dexamfetamine is said to raise the seizure threshold and is usually recommended over methylphenidate, which is said to lower it, in the treatment of *constitutionally* hyperactive children with epilepsy. In practice, methylphenidate may ameliorate or alter the seizure pattern in addition to its expected effect.[171,172]

Anticonvulsants may increase seizure frequency.[173-177] This is more likely to occur where epileptic syndromes are unrecognised or seizure types have not been classified correctly.

Carbamazepine and sodium valproate are used as psychotropic agents in adults who do not have epilepsy, particularly in the treatment of bipolar illness[178] and episodic dyscontrol (see below). The dose range is the same as for epilepsy. Lamotrigine may have a similar psychotropic effect.[83] Sometimes a mental illness superimposed upon epilepsy can be treated by increasing the dose of an anticonvulsant the child is already taking.

Review of children with "known epilepsy" is recommended above; it is also important to consider the possibility of epilepsy in children with behavioural problems who are "known not to have epilepsy".

Behaviour problems following head injury

Acute behavioural problems arising in the intensive care unit after head injury are not discussed here. Post-traumatic seizures are managed if they arise, and prophylactic anticonvulsants are no longer routine. In the majority of children with behavioural sequelae, these will not be sufficiently incapacitating to consider medication. Seven per cent required antidepressants in one series.[179] The tricyclics are best avoided because anticholinergic drugs may have negative effects on memory and motor performance.[10] Explosive behaviour or episodic dyscontrol will often respond to carbamazepine or sodium valproate (see below). Stimulants may be considered for disinhibited "frontal type" behaviour and amantadine likewise, and also for abulia, which is profound passivity and anergia.[10,180]

Behaviour problems in children with learning disabilities

The American usage "mentally retarded" is politically incorrect in the UK, as is "mentally handicapped", and so this chapter mostly uses the locally correct phrase "learning disabled" to refer to the same thing.

Assessment follows the usual lines of history, physical examination (including height, weight, and head circumference plotted on percentile charts), and investigation. The first step is to identify which behaviours are problematic and then choose one and take a proper history. A behavioural history is taken in the same way as a pain history (what, where, when, how long, and how often?; what brings it on?; what makes it better?; what did you do?; what else have you tried?; and so on). Patients with more than one type of pain will usually have separate enquiry made about each pain type, and likewise about each type of problem behaviour. If this type of proper history is completed by a clinical psychologist, it is called a functional analysis.

Of great importance is where the behaviours occur. Dependent children and youngsters are found in a limited range of settings – home, nursery/school, with their peers, and in the clinic. Behaviours that only occur in certain settings are situational and, unless the situation is the home or the clinician's office, additional informants may be required. Situational behavioural problems are best addressed in the setting in which the problems occur, and it would be most unusual to recommend medication. Pervasive problems occur in all settings and are worse, not least because one does not know whether the child is currently able to behave in any other way.

Having decided with parents which unwanted behaviours are to be targeted, baseline frequencies of each type of behaviour should be recorded. This need not be complicated; we use simple diaries with a month to a page, and a day per line. Diaries may need to be kept in more than one setting. Baselines are recorded so that improvement can be assessed later and because some patients improve without further intervention while baselines are being recorded. The occasional patient who naughtily refuses to exhibit the undesired behaviour while it is being counted should be treated with maintenance baseline recording.

For children with recent behavioural deterioration and limited communication ability, consider physical causes (for example, toothache, earache, headache, tummy ache, or foreign bodies) and think of social stresses particularly in looked-after children where nobody may have mentioned that a favourite member of staff has left recently. Specific psychiatric diagnoses, for example depression or bipolar disorder,[181] should also be considered.

Without going into detail, the management of hyperactivity can be used to illustrate these points. Situational hyperactivity, for example at home and not at school, is best managed by behavioural intervention at home and vice versa; drugs are not required. Acute onset hyperactivity should prompt medical assessment and review of any drugs the child may be taking. Pervasive hyperactivity (at home, at school, and in the doctor's office) will lead to consideration of structural adjustments, medication, and, if the child is already medicated, whether that medication is causing it.

The majority of behaviour problems in the young learning disabled population are of the naughty and oppositional type (conduct disorder), situational, and likely to respond to simple behavioural techniques.[22,182,183] Sleep problems are also very common[184] and often respond to behavioural management where this is available. In the UK, the involvement of community learning disability team nurses can be invaluable.

Severe sleep problems are persistent and incapacitating for the whole family.[184] Synthetic melatonin is increasingly the agent chosen for sleep–wake cycle problems. Most studies have been conducted in children who are blind or have neurodevelopmental disorders. Melatonin is given half an hour before bedtime, the fast release preparation for difficulty in settling or the slow release preparation for sleep maintenance. Habituation has been noted and there may be differences in bioavailability between different preparations. If effective, melatonin should be reduced and stopped every few months to check whether it is still required.[185]

Children presenting seriously incapacitating behaviour problems are likely to need multiple interventions, together with an increase in structure. In school this may mean an increased staff : pupil ratio or exclusion; at home the child might require more adult supervision than another child of the same age with normal development.

Children with learning disability who present with *severe* behavioural problems divide conveniently into two groups: on drugs and not on drugs.

On drugs

Those who are on drugs are probably on too many. Treatment comprises drug rationalisation and reduction in the shadow of tardive dyskinesia.[186] One psychoactive drug at a time is a sensible target. Delirium is usually recognised when it occurs but sometimes the fluctuating symptoms of a subacute confusional state are misinterpreted. Fluctuation in consciousness with lucid intervals is a neuropsychiatric ESR (i.e. the neuropsychiatric equivalent of a raised erythrocyte sedimentation rate); it means that something is seriously wrong. Psychomotor behaviour, thinking, memory, perception, and emotions may also be disturbed. Standard paediatric textbooks present a list of the many possible causes of confusion, which include fever, infection, and non-convulsive status epilepticus, as well as drugs.

Any drug prescribed to improve behaviour may make it worse. Medicated children with developmental disability and behaviour problems are particularly at risk for the prescribing cascade that has been reported in the elderly[187]: drug one causes an adverse drug effect that is misinterpreted as a new medical condition; this leads to prescription of drug two, which leads to adverse drug effects; in turn, these lead to prescription of drug three; and so on.

A drug that does not make a difference should be stopped.

Not on drugs

Children and teenagers with learning disability who present with behaviour problems severe enough to warrant consideration of drug treatment will usually have self injurious behaviour or challenging behaviour if they do not have a more conventional diagnosis, for example depression or bipolar disorder,[181] which should be treated appropriately.

Self injurious behaviour, for example head banging or eye gouging, is very difficult to treat; the most useful intervention is likely to be involvement of an interested clinical psychologist. Naltrexone has been tried in recent years with some success,[188,189] but it makes Rett syndrome worse.[190] Carbamazepine[191,192] or clomipramine[193] can also be used.

Challenging behaviour usually refers to explosive and aggressive behaviour in strong teenagers with limited language and limited responsiveness to social cues. It is not an indication for inpatient treatment. Management is chronic. It is expensive, person intensive, and requires structure, continuity, environmental manipulation (sufficient indoor space and a garden), and attention to augmentative communication systems, for example symbol timetables for each segment of the day to avoid surprises.[194] A regular exercise programme may also be of help[195] and some patients like to shelter under a Ball Blanket (Protac I/S, Aarhus, Denmark). Drugs may have a role to play and should always be assessed with a serial record of the frequency of the target behaviours against a baseline taken before the drug was started.

Drug treatment should be considered for children whose behaviour problems are severely incapacitating,[9] for example a boy who will be unable to remain at home unless his behaviour improves. Sometimes the choice may be "on medication and living at home" or "saved from medication and living in a children's home". The latter seems worse.

Some drugs are unavailable to children who will not take tablets.

If psychoactive drugs are to be used, then use low toxicity drugs first and only one at a time.

Neuroleptics, for example haloperidol and risperidone, should be avoided as far as possible because of the risks for withdrawal dyskinesia and tardive dyskinesia[55] that can follow even a short period of neuroleptic treatment at low dose.[13,186] Their reputation is seductive. A recent systematic review found no evidence of their efficacy in learning disabled adults with challenging behaviour.[196] Tardive dyskinesia also remains a risk for the atypical neuroleptics, with which we have less experience.[41]

If a behaviour sounds cyclical, then this should be verified with a diary. Separate trials of carbamazepine[10,87,197] retard, sodium valproate,[87,197–199], and lithium[200] could all be considered, as well as whether the problem is menstruation related.[111,201,202]

In explosive behaviour or episodic dyscontrol, carbamazepine[10,28,197] retard, valproate,[203] or lithium[68,204,205] may be tried. As Gualtieri[10] pointed out, therapeutic trials are hypothesis testing. In explosive behaviour the issue is "Does he respond to carbamazepine?", not "Could this be epilepsy? (then I can give him carbamazepine)".

Stimulants are also effective for pervasive hyperactivity in learning disabled children[206] but less often in those with severe learning disability. This group of children may be more sensitive to stimulant side effects[207] and cognitive over-focusing can be a problem.[162]

If the behaviours appear anxiety driven, then propranolol may be considered[208–210] or one of the tricyclics, for example imipramine or amitriptyline.

Serotonergics (for example, fluoxetine, fluvoxamine, and sertraline) are probably most prominent among the other drugs chosen now, and many would use them first in behaviour problems associated with autism of a severity to require drug treatment.[211] DeLong et al.[212] suggested that serotonergics may improve the core deficits in a subset of children with autism, and hyperlexia, and family history of major affective disorders and unusual intellectual achievement. Serotonergics can also be used in the management of premenstrual syndrome[202] and stereotypies,[193] which may also be helped by a regular exercise programme.[213]

Naltrexone has been used in autism in lower dose and small alterations seem important.[214–216] Its most consistent effect is a reduction in hyperactivity.[210] Fenfluramine had fallen out of favour for autism before it became unavailable because of the risk for pulmonary hypertension.

Children whose challenging behaviour responds to drug treatment without adverse effects should be kept under review. A period without further change to allow everyone to settle down and regroup is sensible. If the child is settled but on a cocktail of drugs, this will need to be rationalised, which can be done slowly, after the settling period, or very slowly if there is a lot of carer anxiety.

Stopping drugs

The duration of drug treatment varies with the condition. Antidepressants are usually continued for about 4–6 months after a response is obtained.[108,109] I do not usually begin medication withdrawal at critical times, for example at the start of the new school year or just before the family holiday. Different drugs have different indications and rates of withdrawal. It might take more than a year to get a child off clobazam or clonazepam that was originally prescribed for epilepsy, which is a good reason to avoid these drugs in the first place. Unless a more specific recommendation is applicable, reduction and stopping over one or two months, or over a series of clinics is common practice. Withdrawal syndromes have been described for many psychotropics, notably the shorter half life serotonergic antidepressants.[15,108] Neuroleptic reduction may cause a withdrawal dyskinesia, which may not be temporary.

Conclusion

It is always a serious decision to recommend that parents give drugs to their children. Sometimes it is a serious omission not to recommend that parents give drugs to their children. In our present state of knowledge, only one psychoactive drug at a time is a sensible aspiration. A summary of the fundamental principles of drug therapy for psychiatric problems in children is presented in Box 10.1.

Box 10.1 Fundamental principles of drug therapy for psychiatric problems in children

Be methodical.
Always consider poor compliance.
Unless limited by side effects, increase each drug until a response is obtained, or up to the usually accepted maximum dosage for size, before deciding that it is unhelpful and reducing and stopping the drug.
A drug that does not make a difference should be stopped.
Any drug prescribed to improve behaviour may make it worse.
Treatment will often comprise drug reduction and rationalisation.
If psychoactive drugs must be used, then choose low toxicity drugs first.
Neuroleptics, for example haloperidol and risperidone, should be avoided as far as possible because of the risk for tardive dyskinesia that can follow even a short period of neuroleptic treatment at low dose.
There is never an indication to use more than one neuroleptic at the same time.
More than one diagnosis is common in child psychiatry; each diagnosis does not need its own tablets.
Only one psychoactive drug at a time is a sensible aspiration in our present state of knowledge.

Acknowledgements

I am grateful to Carolyn Florence for typing the manuscript. The proposals here build upon previous articles.[217,218]

References

1 Jensen PS, Bhatara VS, Vitiello B, Hoagwood K, Feil M, Burke LB. Psychoactive medication prescribing practices for U.S. children: gaps between research and clinical practice. *J Am Acad Child Adolesc Psychiatry* 1999;**38**:557–65.
2 Jensen PS, Kettle L, Roper M, *et al*. Are stimulants over prescribed? Treatment of ADHD in four U.S. communities. *J Am Acad Child Adolesc Psychiatry* 1999;**8**:151–9.
3 Phillips T, Salmon G, James AC. Prescribing practices in child and adolescent psychiatry: change over time 1993–2000. *Child Adolesc Mental Health* 2003;**8**:23–8.
4 McNicholas F. Prescribing practices of child psychiatrists in the U.K. *Child Psychol Psychiatry Rev* 2001;**6**:166–71.
5 AACAP Official Action. Practice parameters for the use of stimulant medication in the treatment of children, adolescents and adults. *J Am Acad Child Adolesc Psychiatry* 2002;**41**:26S–49S.
6 Bramble D. Psychostimulants and British child psychiatrists. *Child Psychol Psychiatry Rev* 1997;**2**:159–62.
7 Adams S. Prescribing of psychotropic drugs to children and adolescents. *BMJ* 1991;**302**:217.
8 Bramble DJ. The use of anti-depressants by British child psychiatrists. *Psychiatr Bull* 1992;**16**:396–8.
9 British Association for Psychopharmacology. Child and learning disability psychopharmacology BAP consensus statement. *J Psychopharmacol* 1997;**11**:291–4.
10 Gualtieri CT. *Neuropsychiatry and behavioral pharmacology*. New York: Springer-Verlag, 1991.
11 Gualtieri CT. *Brain injury and mental retardation. Psychopharmacology and neuropsychiatry*. Philadelphia: Lippincott Williams & Wilkins, 2002.
12 Ratey JJ, ed. *Mental retardation: developing pharmacotherapies*. Washington, DC: American Psychiatric Press, 1991.
13 Green WH. *Child and adolescent clinical psychopharmacology*. Baltimore: Williams and Wilkins, 2001.
14 Arana GW, Rosenbaum JF, eds. *Handbook of psychiatric drug therapy*. Lippincott, Williams & Wilkins: London, 2000.
15 Bazire S. *Psychotropic drug directory. The professionals pocket handbook and aide memoire*. Dinton: Quay Books, 2000.
16 Riddle MA, Kastelic EA, Frosch E. Paediatric psychopharmacology. *J Child Psychol Psychiatry* 2001;**42**:73–90.
17 Santosh PJ, Baird G. Psychopharmacotherapy in children and adults with intellectual disability. *Lancet* 1999;**354**:233–42.
18 Healy D, Nutt D. Prescriptions, licences and evidence. *Psychiatr Bull* 1998;**22**:680–4.
19 RCPCH Medicines for Children. Royal College of Paediatrics and Child Health: London, 1999:xiii–xv.
20 Cooper JR, Bloom FE, Roth RH. *The biochemical basis of neuropharmacology*. New York: Oxford University Press, 1996.
21 Douglas J, Richman N. *My child won't sleep*. Harmondsworth: Penguin, 1988.
22 Patterson GR. *Living with children*. Champagne: Illinois Research Press, 1975.
23 *British National Formulary number 41*. London: British Medical Association and Royal Pharmaceutical Society of Great Britain, 2001.
24 Simonoff EA, Stores G. Controlled trial of trimeprazine tartrate (alimemazine) for night waking. *Arch Dis Child* 1987;**62**:253–7.
25 Parkes JD. *Sleep and its disorders*. London: WB Saunders, 1985.
26 Lask B. Novel and non-toxic treatment for night terrors. *BMJ* 1988;**297**:592.

27 Pesikoff RB, Davis PC. Treatment of pavor nocturnus and somnambulism in children. *Am J Psychiatry* 1971;**128**:778–81.
28 Puente RM. The use of carbamazepine in the treatment of behavioural disorders in children. In: Birkmayer W, ed. *Epileptic seizures, behaviour, pain.* Bern: Hans Huber Publishers, 1976:243–52.
29 Mouret J, Sanches P, Taillard J, Lemoine P, Robelin N, Canini F. Treatment of narcolepsy with L-tyrosine. *Lancet* 1988;**ii**:1458–9.
30 Elwes RC, Chesterman LP, Jenner P, *et al.* Treatment of narcolepsy with L-tyrosine: double-blind placebo controlled trial. *Lancet* 1989;**ii**:1067–9.
31 Winter E, Prendergast M, Green A. Narcolepsy in a two year old boy. *Dev Med Child Neurol* 1996;**38**:356–70.
32 Williams DT. Neuropsychiatric signs, symptoms and syndromes. In: Lewis M, ed. *Child and adolescent psychiatry*, 2nd edn. Baltimore: Williams and Wilkins, 1996.
33 Nelson HE, Trasher S, Barnes TRE. Practical ways of alleviating auditory hallucinations. *BMJ* 1991;**302**:327.
34 Garralda ME. Hallucinations in children with conduct and emotional disorders: 1. The clinical phenomena. *Psychol Med* 1984;**14**:589–96.
35 Garralda ME. Hallucinations in children with conduct and emotional disorders: 2. The follow-up study. *Psychol Med* 1984;**14**:597–604.
36 Campbell M, Rapoport JL, Simpson GM. Antipsychotics in children and adolescents. *J Am Acad Child Adolesc Psychiatry* 1999;**38**:537–45.
37 Clark AF, Lewis SW. Treatment of schizophrenia in childhood and adolescence. *J Child Psychol Psychiatry* 1998;**39**:1071–81.
38 Spencer EK, Campbell M. Children with schizophrenia: diagnosis, phenomenology and pharmacotherapy. *Schizophr Bull* 1994;**20**:713–25.
39 Mandoki M. Risperidone treatment of children and adolescents: increased risk of extrapyramidal side effects? *J Child Adolesc Psychopharmacol* 1995;**5**:49–67.
40 Toren P, Laor N, Weizman A. Use of atypical neuroleptics in child and adolescent psychiatry. *J Clin Psychiatry* 1998;**59**:644–56.
41 Barnes TRE, McPhillps MA. Critical analysis and comparison of the side-effect and safety profiles of the new antipsychotics. *Br J Psychiatry* 1999;**174**(suppl 38):34–43.
42 *Effective Health Care.* Drug treatments for schizophrenia. 1999;**5**:1–12.
43 Kapur S, Remington G. Atypical antipsychotics. *BMJ* 2000;**321**:1360–1.
44 Geddes J, Freemantle N, Harrison P, Bebbington P. Atypical psychotics in the treatment of schizophrenia, systematic overview and meta-regression analysis. *BMJ* 2000;**321**:1371–6.
45 Eggers C, Ropke B. Pharmacotherapy of schizophrenia in childhood and adolescence. In: Eggers C, ed. *Schizophrenia and youth. Etiology and therapeutic consequences.* Berlin: Springer-Verlag, 1991:182–95.
46 Remschmidt H, Schulz E, Matthias Martin PD. An open trial of clozapine in thirty six adolescents with schizophrenia. *J Child Adolesc Psychopharmacology* 1994;**4**:31–41.
47 Kumra S, Frazier JA, Jacobsen LK, *et al.* Childhood-onset schizophrenia. A double-blind clozapine-haloperidol comparison. *Arch Gen Psychiatry* 1996;**53**:1090–7.
48 Ciompi L. Affect logic and schizophrenia. In: Eggers C, ed. *Schizophrenia and youth. Etiology and therapeutic consequences.* Berlin: Springer-Verlag, 1991:20.
49 Boodhoo JA, Sandler M. Anticholinergic antiparkisonian drugs in psychiatry. *Br J Hosp Med* 1991;**46**:167–9.
50 Pall HS, Williams AC, Blake DR. Iron, akathisia and antipsychotic drugs. *Lancet* 1986;**ii**:1469.
51 Kutcher SP, MacKenzie S, Galarraga W, Szalai J. Clonazepam treatment of adolescents with neuroleptic induced akathisia. *Am J Psychiatry* 1987;**144**:823–4.
52 Silva RR, Munoz DM, Alpert M, Perlmutter IR, Diaz J. Neuroleptic malignant syndrome in children and adolescents. *J Am Acad Child Adolesc Psychiatry* 1999;**38**:187–94.
53 Pelonero AL, Levenson JL, Pandurangi AK. Neuroleptic malignant syndrome. In: Joseph AB, Young RR, eds. *Movement disorders in neurology and neuropsychiatry*, 2nd edn. Oxford: Blackwell, 1999:106–14.
54 Wolf DV, Wagner KD. Tardive dyskinesia, tardive dystonia and tardive Tourette's syndrome in children and adolescents. *J Child Adolesc Psychopharmacol* 1993;**3**:175–98.

55 Gualtieri CT, Schroeder SR, Hicks RE, Quade D. Tardive dyskinesia in young mentally retarded individuals. *Arch Gen Psychiatry* 1986;**43**:335–40.
56 Lees AJ. *Tics and related disorders.* Edinburgh: Churchill Livingstone, 1985.
57 Cunningham-Owens DG. Drug related movement disorders. In: Robertson MM, Eapen V, eds. *Movement and allied disorders in childhood.* Chichester: John Wiley & Sons, 1995:199–236.
58 Casey DE. Clozapine: neuroleptic-induced EPS and tardive dyskinesia. *Psychopharmacol* 1989;**99(suppl)**:S47–53.
59 Levkovitch Y, Kronenberg J, Kayser N, *et al.* Clozapine for tardive dyskinesia in adolescents. *Brain Dev* 1995;**17**:213–5.
60 Casey DE. Paradoxical tardive dyskinesia. In: Joseph AB, Young RR, eds. *Movement disorders in neurology and neuropsychiatry,* 2nd edn. Oxford: Blackwell, 1999:58–60.
61 Jankovic J, Beach J. Long-term effects of tetrabenazine in hyperkinetic movement disorders. *Neurology* 1997;**48**:358–62.
62 Adler LA, Rotrosen J, Edson R, *et al.* Vitamin E treatment for tardive dyskinesia. *Arch Gen Psychiatry* 1999;**56**:836–41.
63 Shapiro E, Shapiro AK, Fulop G, *et al.* Controlled study of haloperidol, pimozide and placebo for the treatment of Gilles de la Tourette syndrome. *Arch Gen Psychiatry* 1989;**46**:722–30.
64 Kelly DL, Conley RR, Love RC, Horn DS, Ushchak CM. Weight gain in adolescents treated with risperidone and conventional antipsychotics over six months. *J Child Adolesc Psychopharmacol* 1998;**8**:151–9.
65 Cree A, Shameem M, Fahy T. A review of the treatment options for clozapine-induced hypersalivation. *Psychiatr Bull* 2001;**25**:114–6.
66 McKane JP, Hall C, Akram G. Hyoscine patches in clozapine-induced hypersalivation. *Psychiatr Bull* 2001;**25**:277.
67 Reilly JG, Ayis SA, Ferrier IN, Jones SJ, Thomas SIIL. QTc-interval abnormalities and psychotropic drug therapy in psychiatric patients. *Lancet* 2000; **355**:1048–52.
68 Alessi N, Naylor MW, Ghaziuddin M, Zubieta JK. Update on lithium carbonate therapy in children and adolescents. *J Am Acad Child Adolesc Psychiatry* 1994;**33**:291–304.
69 Kafantaris V. Treatment of bipolar disorder in children and adolescents. *J Am Acad Child Adolesc Psychiatry* 1995;**34**:732–41.
70 James ACD, Javaloyes AM. The treatment of bipolar disorder in children and adolescents. *J Child Psychol Psychiatry* 2001;**42**:439–49.
71 Jefferson JW. Lithium. Still effective despite its detractors. *BMJ* 1998;**316**:1330–1.
72 Anonymous. Using lithium safely. *Drug Ther Bull* 1999;**37**:22–4.
73 Schou M. Effects of long-term lithium treatment on kidney function: an overview. *J Psychiatr Res* 1988;**22**:287–96.
74 Waller DG, Edwards JG. Lithium and the kidney: an update. *Psychol Med* 1989;**19**:825–31.
75 Ferrier IN, Tyrer SP, Bell AJ. Lithium therapy. *Adv Psychiatr Treat* 1995;**1**:102–10.
76 Bendz H, Sjödin I, Toss G, Berglund K. Hyperparathyroidism and long-term lithium therapy: a cross-sectional study and the effect of lithium withdrawal. *J Intern Med* 1996;**240**:357–65.
77 Calabrese JR, Kimmel SE, Woyshville MJ, *et al.* Clozapine for treatment-refractory mania. *Am J Psychiatry* 1996; **153(suppl 3)**:759–64.
78 Kowatch RA, Suppes T, Gilfillan SK, Fuentes RM, Grannemann BD, Emslie GJ. Clozapine treatment of children and adolescents with bipolar disorder and schizophrenia: a clinical case series. *J Child Adolesc Psychopharmacol* 1995;**5**: 241–53.
79 Ryan ND, Bhatara VS, Perel JM. Mood stabilizers in children and adolescents. *J Am Acad Child Adolesc Psychiatry* 1999;**38**:529–36.
80 Kowatch RA, Suppes T, Carmody TJ, *et al.* Effect size of lithium, divalproex sodium and carbamazepine in children and adolescents with bipolar disorder. *J Am Acad Child Adolesc Psychiatry* 2000;**39**:713–20.
81 Papatheodorou G, Kutcher SP, Katic M, Szalai JP. The efficacy and safety of divalproex sodium in the treatment of acute mania in adolescents and young adults: an open clinical trial. *J Clin Psychopharmacol* 1995;**15**:110–6.
82 West SA, Keck PE, McElroy SL, *et al.* Open trial of valproate in the treatment of adolescent mania. *J Child Adolesc Psychopharmacol* 1994;**4**:263–7.

83   Duncan D, McConnell HW, Taylor D. Lamotrigine in bipolar affective disorder. *Psychiatr Bull* 1998;**22**:630–2.
84   Sporn J, Sachs G. The anticonvulsant lamotrigine in treatment-resistant manic-depressive illness. *J Clin Psychopharmacol* 1997;**17**:185–9.
85   Bauer MS, Whybrow PC, Winokur A. Rapid cycling bipolar affective disorder in association with grade 1 hypothyroidism. *Arch Gen Psychiatry* 1990;**47**:427–32.
86   Pollard AJ, Prendergast M, Al-Hamouri F, Rayner PW, Shaw NJ. Different subtypes of pseudo hypoparathyroidism in the same family with an unusual psychiatric presentation of the index case. *Arch Dis Child* 1994;**70**:90–102.
87   Taylor D, Duncan D. Treatment options for rapid-cycling bipolar affective disorder. *Psychiatr Bull* 1996;**20**:601–3.
88   Calabrese JR, Woyshville MJ. A medication algorithm for treatment of bipolar rapid cycling? *J Clin Psychiatry* 1995;**56(suppl 3)**:11–8.
89   Kusumakar V, Yatham LN, Haslam DRS, *et al.* Treatment of mania, mixed state and rapid cycling. *Can J Psychiatry* 1997;**42(suppl 2)**:79S–86S.
90   Wright EC. Non-compliance – or how many aunts has Matilda? *Lancet* 1993;**342**:909–13.
91   Yamashita I. Periodic psychosis of adolescence. Hokkaido University Press, 1993.
92   Jayson D, Wood A, Kroll L, Fraser J, Harrington R. Which depressed patients respond to cognitive behaviour therapy? *J Am Acad Child Adolesc Psychiatry* 1998;**37**:35–9.
93   Harrington R. Depressive disorder in childhood and adolescence. Chichester: Wiley & Sons, 1993.
94   Emslie GJ, Rush AJ, Weinberg WA, *et al.* A double-blind, randomised, placebo-controlled trial of fluoxetine in children and adolescents with depression. *Arch Gen Psychiatry* 1997;**54**:1031–7.
95   Emslie GJ, Walkup JT, Pliszka SR, Ernst M. Nontricyclic antidepressants: current trends in children and adolescents. *J Am Acad Child Adolesc Psychiatry* 1999;**38**:517–28.
96   Coulter DM, Pillans PI. Fluoxetine and extrapyramidal side effects. *Am J Psychiatry* 1995;**152**:122–5.
97   Budman CL, Bruun RD. Persistent dyskinesia in a patient receiving fluoxetine. *Am J Psychiatry* 1991;**148**:1403.
98   Jones-Fearing KB. SSRI and EPS with fluoxetine. *J Am Acad Child Adolesc Psychiatry* 1996;**35**:1107–8.
99   Bernstein JG. Serotonin syndrome. In: Joseph AB, Young RR, eds. *Movement disorders in neurology and neuropsychiatry*, 2nd edn. Oxford: Blackwell, 1999: 426–33.
100   Mir S, Taylor D. Serotonin syndrome. *Psychiatr Bull* 1999;**23**:742–7.
101   Spirko BA, Wiley JF. Serotonin syndrome: a new pediatric intoxication. *Pediatr Emerg Care* 1999;**15**:440–3.
102   Achamallah NS, Decker DH. Mania induced by fluoxetine in an adolescent patient. *Am J Psychiatry* 1991;**148**:1404.
103   Briscoe JJD, Harrington RC, Prendergast M. Development of mania in close association with tricyclic anti-depressant administration in children. *Eur Child Adolesc Psychiatry* 1995;**4**:280–3.
104   James AC. Case report: mixed mania: apparent induction in an adolescent by a selective serotonin reuptake inhibitor antidepressant (SSRI). *Clin Child Psychol Psychiatry* 1996;**1**:621–4.
105   Hughes CW, Emslie GJ, Crismon ML, *et al.* The Texas children's medication algorithm project: report of the Texas consensus conference panel on medication treatment of childhood major depressive disorder. *J Am Acad Child Adolesc Psychiatry* 1999;**38**:1442–54.
106   Geller B, Reising D, Leonard HL, Riddle MA, Walsh BT. Critical review of tricyclic antidepressant use in children and adolescents. *J Am Acad Child Adolesc Psychiatry* 1999;**38**:513–6.
107   Puig-Antich J, Perel JM, Lupatkin W, *et al.* Imipramine in pre-pubertal major depressive disorders. *Arch Gen Psychiatry* 1987;**44**:81–9.
108   Anonymous. Withdrawing patients from antidepressants. *Drug Ther Bull* 1999;**37**:49–52.

109 Anderson IM, Nutt DJ, Deakin JFW. Evidence-based guidelines for treating depressive disorders with antidepressants: a revision of the 1993 British Association for Psychopharmacology guidelines. *J Psychopharmacol* 2000;**14**:3–20.
110 Giles H. Imipramine poisoning in childhood. *BMJ* 1963;**ii**:844–6.
111 Leibenluft B, Wehr TA. Is sleep deprivation useful in the treatment of depression? *Am J Psychiatry* 1992;**149**:159–68.
112 King BH, Baxter LR, Stuber M, Fish B. Therapeutic sleep deprivation for depression in children. *J Am Acad Child Adolesc Psychiatry* 1987;**26**:928–31.
113 Naylor MW, King CA, Lindsay KA, *et al.* Sleep deprivation in depressed adolescents and psychiatric controls. *J Am Acad Child Adolesc Psychiatry* 1993;**32**:753–9.
114 Swedo SE, Allen AJ, Glod CA, *et al.* A controlled trial of light therapy for the treatment of pediatric seasonal affective disorder. *J Am Acad Child Adolesc Psychiatry* 1997;**36**:816–21.
115 Saha S, Pariante CM, McArdle TF, Fombonne E. Very early onset seasonal affective disorder: a case study. *Eur Child Adolesc Psychiatry* 2000;**9**:135–8.
116 Meesters YBE. Case study: dawn simulation as maintenance treatment in a nine year-old patient with seasonal affective disorder. *J Am Acad Child Adolesc Psychiatry* 1998;**37**:986–98.
117 Fink M. Catatonia. In: Trimble MR, Cummings JL, eds. *Contemporary behavioural neurology*. Boston: Butterworth-Heinemann, 1997:289–309.
118 Bertagnoli MW, Borchardt CM. A review of ECT for children and adolescents. *J Am Acad Child Adolesc Psychiatry* 1990;**29**:302–7.
119 Flament MF, Rapoport JL, Berg CJ, *et al.* Clomipramine treatment of childhood obsessive compulsive disorder. *Arch Gen Psychiatry* 1985;**42**:977–83.
120 DeVeaugh-Geiss J, Moroz G, Biederman J, *et al.* Clomipramine hydrochloride in children and adolescent obsessive compulsive disorder – a multicentre trial. *J Am Acad Child Adolesc Psychiatry* 1992;**31**:45–9.
121 Riddle MA, Scahill L, King RA, *et al.* Double-blind, crossover trial of fluoxetine and placebo in children and adolescents with obsessive-compulsive disorder. *J Am Acad Child Adolesc Psychiatry* 1992;**31**:1062–9.
122 March JS, Biederman J, Wolkow R, *et al.* Sertraline in children and adolescents with obsessive-compulsive disorder. A multicenter randomized controlled trial. *JAMA* 1998;**280**:1752–6.
123 Swedo SE, Rapoport JL. Trichotillomania. *J Child Psychol Psychiatry* 1991;**32**:401–9.
124 Bruun RD. Subtle and under-recognised side effects of neuroleptic treatment in children with Tourette's disorder. *Am J Psychiatry* 1988;**145**:621–4.
125 Sallee FR, Nesbitt L, Jackson C, Sine L, Sethuraman G. Relative efficacy of haloperidol and pimozide in children and adolescents with Tourette's Disorder. *Am J Psychiatry* 1997;**154**:1057–62.
126 Robertson MM, Schnieden V, Lees AJ. Management of Gilles de la Tourette syndrome using sulpiride. *Clin Neuropharmacol* 1990;**13**:229–35.
127 Singer HS, Gammon K, Quaskey S. Haloperidol, fluphenazine and clonidine in Tourette syndrome: controversies in treatment. *Pediatr Neurosci* 1986;**12**:71–4.
128 Goetz CG, Tanner CM, Klawans HL. Fluphenazine and multifocal tic disorders. *Arch Neurol* 1984;**41**:271–2.
129 Lombroso PJ, Scahill L, King RA, *et al.* Risperidone treatment of children and adolescents with chronic tic disorders: a preliminary report. *J Am Acad Child Adolesc Psychiatry* 1995;**34**:1147–52.
130 Robertson MM, Scull DA, Eapen V, Trimble M. Risperidone in the treatment of Tourette syndrome: a retrospective case note study. *J Psychopharmacol* 1996;**10**:317–20.
131 Silva RR, Magee HJ, Friedhoff AJ. Persistent tardive dyskinesia and other neuroleptic related dyskinesias in Tourette's disorder. *J Child Adolesc Psychopharmacol* 1993;**3**:137–44.
132 Durson SM, Reveley MA, Bird R, Stirton F. Longlasting improvement of Tourette's syndrome with transdermal nicotine. *Lancet* 1994;**344**:1577.
133 Walkup JT, Labellarte MJ, Riddle MA, *et al.* Fluvoxamine for the treatment of anxiety disorders in children and adolescents. *N Engl J Med* 2001;**344**:1279–85.
134 Livingston MG. Interactions with selective MAOIs. *Lancet* 1995;**345**:533–4.

135 Perry C, Jacobs D. Overview: clinical applications of the amytal interview in psychiatry emergency settings. *Am J Psychiatry* 1982;**139**:552–9.

136 White A, Corbin DOC, Coope B. The use of thiopentone in the treatment of non-organic locomotor disorders. *J Psychosom Res* 1988;**32**:249–53.

137 Jimerson DC, Wolfe BE, Brotman A, *et al*. Medication in the treatment of eating disorders. *Psychiatr Clin North Am* 1996;**19**:739–54.

138 Anonymous. Drug treatment of neuropathic pain. *Drug Ther Bull* 2000;**38**:89–93.

139 Clayden GS. Management of chronic constipation. *Arch Dis Child* 1992;**67**:340–4.

140 Elawad MA, Sullivan P. Management of constipation in children with disabilities. *Dev Med Child Neurol* 2001;**43**:829–32.

141 Panayiotopoulos CP. Nocturnal enuresis associated with sodium valproate. *Lancet* 1985;**1**:980–1.

142 Fordham KE, Meadow SR. Controlled study of standard pad and bell alarm against mini alarm for nocturnal enuresis. *Arch Dis Child* 1989;**64**:651–6.

143 Evans JHC, Meadow SR. Desmopressin for bed wetting: length of treatment, vasopressin secretion, and response. *Arch Dis Child* 1992;**67**:184–8.

144 Hourihane J, Salisbury AJ. Use caution in prescribing desmopressin for nocturnal enuresis. *BMJ* 1993;**306**:1545.

145 World Health Organisation. *The ICD-10 classification of mental and behavioural disorders & diagnostic guidelines*. Geneva: WHO, 1992.

146 American Psychiatric Association. *Diagnostic and statistical manual of mental disorders (DSM-IV-TR)*, 4th edn, text revised. Washington, DC: American Psychiatric Association, 2000.

147 Taylor E, Sandberg S, Thorley G, Giles S. *The epidemiology of childhood hyperactivity*. Institute of Psychiatry Maudsley Monographs. London: Oxford University Press, 1991.

148 Prendergast M, Taylor E, Rapoport JL, *et al*. The diagnosis of childhood hyperactivity: a US-UK cross national study of DSM-III and ICD-9. *J Child Psychol Psychiatry* 1988;**29**:289–300.

149 MTA Co-operative Group. A 14 month randomised clinical trial of treatment strategies for attention-deficit/hyperactivity disorder. *Arch Gen Psychiatry* 1999;**56**:1073–86.

150 Greenhill LL, Haperin JM, Abikoff H. Stimulant medications. *J Am Acad Child Adolesc Psychiatry* 1999;**38**:503–12.

151 Taylor E, Sergeant J, Doepfner M, *et al*. Clinical guidelines for hyperkinetic disorder. *Eur Child Adolesc Psychiatry* 1998;**7**:184–200.

152 Foreman DM, Foreman D, Prendergast M, Minty B. The use of screening instruments alter the rate of diagnosis of hyperactivity in a clinic sample of children. A case note study using ICD-10 diagnosis. *Eur Child Adolesc Psychiatry* 2001;**10**:130–4.

153 Rutter M, Tizard J, Whitmore K, eds. *Education, health and behaviour*. London: Longmans Green, 1970.

154 Goyette CH, Conners CK, Ulrich RF. Normative data on revised parent and teacher rating scales. *J Abnorm Child Psychol* 1978;**6**:221–36.

155 Taylor E, Schachar R, Thorley G, Wieselberg HM, Everitt B, Rutter M. Which boys respond to stimulant medication? A controlled trial of methylphenidate in boys with disruptive behaviour. *Psychol Med* 1987;**17**:121–43.

156 Schachar R, Taylor E, Wieselberg M, Thorley G, Rutter M. Changes in family function and relationships in children who respond to methylphenidate. *J Am Acad Child Adolesc Psychiatry* 1987;**26**:728–32.

157 Koizumi HM. Obsessive–compulsive symptoms following stimulants. *Biol Psychiatry* 1985;**20**:1332–3.

158 Borcherding BG, Keysor CS, Rapoport JL, Ammas J. Motor/vocal tics and compulsive behaviours on stimulant drugs: is there a common vulnerability? *Psychiatry Res* 1990;**33**:83–94.

159 Law SF, Schachar RJ. Do typical clinical doses of methylphenidate cause tics in children treated for attention deficit hyperactivity disorder? *J Am Acad Child Adolesc Psychiatry* 1999;**38**:944–51.

160 Ford T, Taylor E, Warner-Rogers J. Sustained release methylphenidate. *Child Psychol Psychiatry Rev* 2000;**5**:108–13.

161 Rapoport JL, Quinn PO, Bradbard G, Riddle D, Brookes E. Imipramine and methylphenidate treatments of hyperactive boys: a double-blind comparison. *Arch Gen Psychiatry* 1974;**30**:789–93.
162 Popper CW. Pharmacologic alternatives to psychostimulants for the treatment of attention-deficit/hyperactivity disorder. *Child Adolesc Clin North Am* 2000;**9**:605–46.
163 Silva RR, Munoz DM, Alpert M. Carbamazepine use in children and adolescents with features of attention deficit hyperactivity disorder: a meta analysis. *J Am Acad Child Adolesc Psychiatry* 1996;**35**:352–8.
164 Connor DF, Fletcher KE, Swanson JM. A meta-analysis of clonidine for symptoms of attention-deficit/hyperactivity disorder. *J Am Acad Child Adolesc Psychiatry* 1999;**38**:1551–9.
165 Scahill L, Chappell PB, Kim YS, Schultz RT, *et al.* A placebo-controlled study of guanfacine in the treatment of children with tic disorders and attention-deficit/hyperactivity disorder. *Am J Psychiatry* 2001;**158**:1067–74.
166 Barrickman LL, Perry PJ, Allen AJ, *et al.* Bupropion versus methylphenidate in the treatment of attention-deficit/hyperactivity disorder. *J Am Acad Child Adolesc Psychiatry* 1995;**34**:649–57.
167 Besag FMC. Behavioural effects of the new anticonvulsants. *Drug Safety* 2001;**24**:513–36.
168 Ryan SW, Forsythe I, Hartley R, Haworth M, Bowmer CJ. Slow release carbamazepine in treatment of poorly controlled seizures. *Arch Dis Child* 1990;**65**:930–5.
169 Stephenson JBP, King MD. *Handbook of neurological investigations in children.* London: Wright, 1989.
170 Commander M, Green SH, Prendergast M. Behavioural disturbances in children treated with clonazepam. *Dev Med Child Neurol* 1991;**33**:362–3.
171 Feldman H, Crumrine P, Handen RL, Alvin R, Teodori J. Methylphenidate in children with seizures and attention deficit disorder. *Am J Dis Children* 1989;**143**:1081–6.
172 Gross-Tsur V, Manor O, van der Meere J, Joseph A, Shalev RS. Epilepsy and attention deficit hyperactivity disorder: is methylphenidate safe and effective? *J Paediatr* 1997;**130**:40–4.
173 Lerman P. Seizures induced or aggravated by anticonvulsants. *Epilepsia* 1986;**27**:706–10.
174 Talwar D, Arora MS, Sher PK. EEG changes and exacerbation in young children treated with carbamazepine. *Epilepsia* 1994;**35**:1154–9.
175 Perucca E, Gram L, Avanzini G, Dulac O. Antiepileptic drugs as a cause of worsening seizures. *Epilepsia* 1998;**39**:5–17.
176 Guerrini R, Dravet C, Genton P, Belmonte A, Kaminska A, Dulac O. Lamotrigine and seizure aggravation in severe myoclonic epilepsy. *Epilepsia* 1998;**39**:508–12.
177 Guerrini R, Belmonte A, Genton P. Antiepileptic drug-induced worsening of seizures in children. *Epilepsia* 1998;**39(suppl 3)**:S2–10.
178 Taylor D, Duncan D. Doses of carbamazepine and valproate in bipolar affective disorder. *Psychiatr Bull* 1997;**21**:224–6.
179 O'Brien G, Cheesebrough B. Traumatic brain damage In: Gillberg C, O'Brien G, eds. *Developmental disability & behaviour.* Clinics in Developmental Medicine 149. Cambridge: MacKeith Press, 2000:64–76.
180 Nickels JL, Schneider WN, Dombovy ML, Wong TM. Clinical use of amantadine in brain injury rehabilitation. *Brain Injury* 1994;**8**:709–18.
181 McCracken JT, Diamond RP. Bipolar disorder in mentally retarded adolescents. *J Am Acad Child Adolesc Psychiatry* 1988;**27**:494–9.
182 Carr J. Helping your handicapped child. Harmondsworth: Penguin, 1995.
183 Howlin P, ed. *Behavioural approaches to problems in childhood.* Clinics in Developmental Medicine 146. Cambridge: MacKeith Press, 1998.
184 Quine L. Sleep problems in children with mental handicap. *J Ment Defic Res* 1991;**35**:269–90.
185 Jan JE, Freeman RD, Fast DK. Melatonin treatment of sleep-wake cycle disorders in children and adolescents. *Dev Med Child Neurol* 1999;**41**:491–500.
186 Campbell M, Armenteros JL, Malone RP, Adams PB, Eisenberg ZW, Overall JE. Neuroleptic related dyskinesias in autistic children: a prospective longitudinal study. *J Am Acad Child Adolesc Psychiatry* 1997;**36**:835–43.

187 Rochon PA, Gurwitz JH. Optimising drug treatment for elderly people: the prescribing cascade. *BMJ* 1997;**315**:1096–9.
188 Barrett RP, Feinstein C, Hole WT. Effects of naloxone and naltrexone on self injury: a double blind placebo controlled analysis. *Am J Ment Retard* 1989;**93**:644–51.
189 Buzan RD, Thomas M, Dubovsky SL, Treadway J. The use of opiate antagonists for recurrent self-injurious behaviour. *J Neuropsychiatry Clin Neurosci* 1995;**7**: 437–44.
190 Percy A, Glaze D, Schultz R, *et al*. Rett syndrome: controlled study of an oral opiate antagonist, naltrexone. *Ann Neurol* 1994;**35**:464–70.
191 Barrett RP, Payton JB, Burkhart JE. Treatment of self injury and disruptive behaviour with carbamazepine (Tegretol) and behaviour therapy. *J Multi-handicapped Person* 1988;**1**:79–91.
192 Roach ES, Delgado M, Anderson L, Iannaccone ST, Burns DK. Carbamazepine trial for Lesch-Nyhan self-mutilation. *J Child Neurol* 1996;**11**:476–8.
193 Garber HJ, McGonigle JJ, Slomka GT, Monteverde E. Clomipramine treatment of stereotypic behaviours and self-injury in patients with developmental disabilities. *J Am Acad Child Adolesc Psychiatry* 1992;**31**:1157–60.
194 Howlin P. Autism. In: *Behavioural approaches in childhood*. Clinics in Developmental Medicine 146. Cambridge: MacKeith Press, 1998.
195 McGimsey JF, Favell JE. The effects of increased physical exercise on disruptive behaviour in retarded persons. *J Autism Dev Disord* 1988;**18**:167–79.
196 Brylewski J, Duggan L. Antipsychotic medication for challenging behaviour in people with intellectual disability: a systematic review of randomized controlled trials. *J Intellect Disabil Res* 1999;**43**:360–71.
197 Sovner R. Use of anticonvulsant agents for the treatment of neuropsychiatric disorders in the developmentally disabled. In: Ratey JJ, ed. *Mental retardation: developing pharmacotherapies*. Washington, DC: American Psychiatric Press, 1991:83–106.
198 Kastner T, Friedman DL, Plummer AT, Ruiz MQ, Henning D. Valproic acid for the treatment of children with mental retardation and mood symptomatology. *Pediatrics* 1990;**86**:467–72.
199 Whittier MC, West SA, Galli VB, Raute NJ. Valproic acid for dysphoric mania in a mentally retarded adolescent. *J Clin Psychiatry* 1995;**56**:590–1.
200 Vanstraelen M, Tyrer SP. Rapid cycling bipolar affective disorder in people with intellectual disability: a systematic review. *J Intellect Disabil Res* 1999;**43**: 349–59.
201 Berga SL. Understanding premenstrual syndrome. *Lancet* 1998;**351**:465.
202 Dimmock PW, Wyatt KM, Jones PW, O'Brien PMS. Efficacy of selective serotonin-reuptake inhibitors in premenstrual syndrome: a systematic review. *Lancet* 2000;**356**:1131–6.
203 Donovan SJ, Stewart JW, Nunes EV, *et al*. Divalproex treatment of youth with explosive temper and mood lability: a double-blind, placebo-controlled crossover design. *Am J Psychiatry* 2000;**157**:818–20.
204 DeLong GR, Aldershof AL. Long-term experience with lithium treatment in childhood: correlation with clinical diagnosis. *J Am Acad Child Adolesc Psychiatry* 1987;**26**:389–94.
205 Tyrer SP, Walsh A, Edwards DE, Berney TP, Stephens DA. Factors associated with a good response to lithium in aggressive mentally handicapped subjects. *Prog Neuropsychopharmacol* 1984;**8**:751–5.
206 Handen BL, Breaux AM, Gosling A, *et al*. Efficacy of methylphenidate among mentally retarded children with attention-deficit/hyperactivity disorder. *Pediatrics* 1990;**86**:922–30.
207 Handen BL, Feldman H, Gosling A, Breaux AM, McAuliffe S. Adverse side effects of methylphenidate among mentally retarded children with ADHD. *J Am Acad Child Adolesc Psychiatry* 1991;**30**:241–5.
208 Ratey JJ, Lindem KJ. Beta blockers as primary treatment for aggression and self injury in the developmentally disabled. In: Ratey JJ, ed. *Mental retardation: developing pharmacotherapies*. Washington, DC: American Psychiatric Press, 1991:51–81.

209 Williams DT, Mehl R, Yudofsky S, Adams D, Roseman B. The effect of propranolol on uncontrolled rage outbursts in children and adolescents with organic brain dysfunction. *J Am Acad Child Psychiatry* 1982;**21**:129–35.
210 Riddle MA, Bernstein GA, Cook EH, Leonard HL, March JS, Swanson JM. Anxiolytics, adrenergic agents, and naltrexone. *J Am Acad Child Adolesc Psychiatry* 1999;**38**:546–56.
211 Cook EH, Rowlett R, Jaselskis C, Leventhal BL. Fluoxetine treatment of children and adults with autistic disorder and mental retardation. *J Am Acad Child Adolesc Psychiatry* 1992;**31**:739–45.
212 DeLong GR, Ritch CR, Burch S. Fluoxetine response in children with autistic spectrum disorders: correlation with familial major affective disorder and intellectual achievement. *Dev Med Child Neurol* 2002;**44**:652–9.
213 Kern L, Koegel RL, Dyer K, Blew PA, Fenton LR. The effects of physical exercise on self-stimulation and appropriate responding in autistic children. *J Autism Dev Disorders* 1982;**4**:399–419.
214 Leboyer M, Bouvard MP, Launay JM, *et al.* A double-blind study of naltrexone in infantile autism. *J Autism Dev Disord* 1992;**22**:309–19.
215 Kolmen BK, Feldman HM, Handen BL, Janosky JE. Naltrexone in young autistic children: replication study and learning measures. *J Am Acad Child Adolesc Psychiatry* 1997;**36**:1570–8.
216 Willemsen-Swinkels SHN, Buitelaar JK, Weijnen FG, van Engeland H. Placebo-controlled acute dosage naltrexone study in young autistic children. *Psychiatry Res* 1995;**58**:203–15.
217 Prendergast M. Types of psychiatric treatment: drug treatment. *Arch Dis Child* 1992;**67**:1488–94.
218 Prendergast M. A pragmatic approach to medication. In: Gillberg C, O'Brien G, eds. *Developmental disability & behaviour*. Clinics in Developmental Medicine 149. Cambridge: MacKeith Press, 2000.

Section III
Working with others

11: Working in primary care

MARGARET JJ THOMPSON

Overview

Behaviour and emotional problems in children are an increasing concern to parents, schools, and society.

Research has indicated that problems of aggression, hyperactivity, and extremes of temper do not go away.

Depression occurs in 1–2% of adolescents, and if not treated it may well recur.

Only the most severe problems are referred into specialised child mental health services (around 10–20% of all problems).

Most emotional and behaviour problems will present in primary care.

Many families would prefer to be offered advice by professionals they know.

The skills of professionals within primary care could be further enhanced to enable them to treat many of these problems themselves.

This support could come from mental health professionals as well as other professionals.

Because resources are tight, Specialist Child and Adolescent Mental Health Services (SCAMHS) must be used creatively.

Introduction

About one in ten children and young people aged five to sixteen years will have an emotional or behavioural problem at any one time that causes them or others concern for their functioning or wellbeing. However, at most only one in five of those will be known to Specialist Child and Adolescent Mental Health Services (SCAMHS).[1]

Many children with such problems will be known to staff in schools, teachers, educational welfare officers or educational psychologists, or to school nurses or community paediatricians. Other staff who work in primary medical services, for example health visitors, general practitioners, or practice counsellors, or in social services may also encounter these young people or their families. It therefore makes sense for primary care staff to develop skills to recognise and treat such problems as soon as they present. Families could then be treated in their own environment. This chapter outlines recent work in this area.

Documents from the Department of Health[2-5] and from the British Paediatric Association[6] have confirmed the need to develop further the skills of primary care teams in the care of mental health. Better partnership between the primary care sector, education and social services, and with secondary care colleagues such as paediatricians and child psychiatrists was encouraged.

The report from the Health Advisory Service[2] delineated a "tier system" for delivery of children's mental health services (Box 11.1). Staff in primary care settings have become known as "tier one services".

Box 11.1 Proposed tier system[2]

Tier one. This is the first line service of non-specialist primary care workers such as school nurses, health visitors, general practitioners, teachers, social workers, and educational welfare officers. Problems seen at this level would be the common ones of childhood: sleeping, feeding, temper tantrums, parent–child interaction, behaviour problems at home and at school, and bereavement.

Tier two. Specialised mental health workers working relatively independently from other services, taking referrals and providing support to primary care colleagues. If appropriate they will offer assessment and treatment in primary care (i.e. family work, bereavement, drop-in groups for parents, parenting groups, and programmes for behaviour problems and anger management). Educational psychologists or clinical psychologists might operate at this level, as would primary mental health workers, who would also mediate between the primary care level and tier three, acting both as a bridge and a filter.

Tier three would consist of multidisciplinary teams who work in specialised CAMHS. Problems seen here would be too complicated to be dealt with at tier two, for example assessment of developmental problems, including autism, hyperactivity, depression, self harm, early psychosis, and severe eating disorders.

Tier four consists of specialised day and inpatient units in which patients with more severe mental illness could be assessed and treated, as well as specialised outpatient services.

General principles

Health visitors and general practitioners are ideally placed to identify problems in families because both see most families with young children and most are still doing developmental checks at six weeks, eighteen months, and three years of age. Many families will present to health workers, and professionals should be prepared to ask the questions behind the presenting symptom, which may reveal depression in the mother or a behaviour or emotional problem in the child.

With training and support from other professionals, health visitors can run groups for mothers with postnatal depression and antenatal and postnatal groups to discuss positive parenting principles. Behavioural techniques have been developed for dealing with behaviour problems, for example sleep and eating difficulties. Many health visitors with their nursery nurses are running behaviour clinics in the community, and these are often supported by staff from SCAMHS.

Parenting work with parents with children with more severe conduct disorder and hyperactivity can be carried out in the community with further training and support or with joint working. Parenting groups in schools are possible; nurturing groups for children who are finding it hard to cope with life in school have been successful; and school nurses can run "drop-in groups" for schools.

Working with general practitioners to aid them in the diagnosis of depression in adolescents has increased their competence with this tricky group of young people who do not like coming to clinics. Primary mental health workers (PMHWs) can help bridge the gap between primary care and SCAMHS. Aspects of this work are described here.

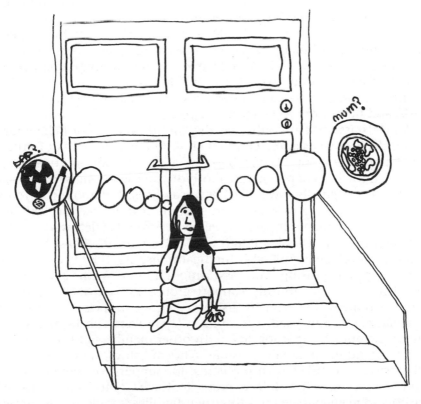

"Who to live with?" Psychiatrists may help other services attend to the needs of children in disturbing situations

Applications as conducted in the clinical locality of the author

Work by health visitors in recognising and assessing young children with behavioural problems

Alongside community health colleagues, the SCAMHS in our locality has developed a service for young children in our clinical area. A questionnaire survey indicated that health visitors thought that they had inadequate background training in the assessment and treatment of preschool children with behavioural problems, but realised that this was an important part of their workload.[7] Initially, single day workshops on sleep problems and postnatal depression were offered. Gradually, however, this evolved into a seven day course, which integrated work with young children and school age children in order to cater for the needs of health visitors, school nurses, and other professionals working with children with mental health problems, because in our area school nurses and health visitors are becoming more generic in their approach. To accompany the theoretical aspects of the course, two manuals were produced that gave practical advice to primary health workers, social workers, community paediatricians, and teachers on how to tackle problems within their setting. The course was practice based and was delivered in two blocks in order for tasks and homework to be set in between.[8,9]

A needs assessment confirmed that the prevalence of behavioural problems in three year old children (13.4%) was as high in our urban/rural population[10] as it had been in a urban community study,[11] although the level of psychiatric morbidity in the mothers in the rural study was marginally lower (27.1% versus 30%). A random controlled trial of the delivery of a sleep programme to non-sleeping children aged 2–4 years and their parents was successful.[12] Leaflets were written for parents of preschool children with behaviour problems.[13–17]

As we developed work with the health visitors, they became more skilled in recognising and assessing children with behavioural problems. We ran monthly support groups in each locality, which were attended by health visitors, school nurses, community paediatricians, and paediatric nurses. These were run by the senior nurse therapist for that locality, with other members of the SCAMHS team attending if at all possible. The meetings were used for a discussion of families with problems, for support for ongoing work, and discussion of possible referrals to the SCAMHS clinic. Health visitors were encouraged to bring their families for a joint assessment at the clinic, which meant that health visitors could see our team in action and observe another way of looking at the problem, while also helping to validate their work with families, because families often misperceived health visitors as not having the necessary skills.[7,18] Referrals from health visitors were very low when the author started in the clinic in 1984 (eight per year; 6% of clinic referrals). This rose to 120 per year in 1994 (25% of clinic referrals), but referrals have gradually fallen as the health visitors have become more skilled and able to deal with the simpler problems themselves (50 referrals during the year 2001; 9% of clinic referrals).

A community health visitor screening programme for hyperactivity

With the support of the health visitors, we undertook a screening programme for hyperactivity in the community and from that we developed a parenting package for parents of hyper-active three year old children. This package was delivered by nurses operating at tier two, with 53% of the families improving to preclinical levels.[19] With further research funding, we were able to train health visitors in the community to determine whether this package was generalisable to tier one professionals. The health visitors found the package easy to use, and they and the families both liked the package, but the results were less good, with only 27% of families improving. We believe that the reason for this was that the health visitors had less time to devote to the work and make use of available supervision because of high case loads, even though their time had been "bought out".[20]

The families who had the intervention are being followed up currently to determine the influence of the package on the future behaviour and referral patterns of the children. Bearing in mind that hyperactivity can have a major influence on a child's future wellbeing and conduct, this follow up is important.

Child and Adolescent Mental Health Service nurses running community clinics

Our work in the community was developed further, with SCAMHS nurses working as primary mental health nurses for about half of their time, seeing families and running community clinics on their own (tier two work). We costed this different service recently and found that these clinics cost about three-fifths that of the previous service operating in tier three, with little difference in the effect size (2.5/2.1).[21]

Since that time, some of the health visitors have decided to take the work further and have set up their own behavioural clinics with the support of our SCAMHS. Most health visitors have nursery nurses working with them, and they are undertaking the behaviour packages supervised by the health visitors. Recently, the SCAMHS has also been running a support group specifically for nursery nurses.

Case example: a difficult three year old

A health visitor spoke to our senior nurse therapist about a Mrs Smith whose three year old was extremely difficult to cope with at playgroup. The playgroup leaders had said that she was distractible, was not concentrating, and had difficulties playing with other children. Our nurse therapist discussed with the health visitor the assessment of the child's difficulties, and the Routh Activity Scale[22] (an adaption of the Werry–Weis scale – a 27 item checklist for overactive behaviours suitable for use in community settings that is easy to score) indicated that the child was highly active. On the temperament scale, it was clear that she had a labile temperament with a high score for emotionality (EAS temperament scale[23] – a 20 item scale, of which we use only the emotionality and shyness subscales; health visitors find it easy to use).

Our nurse therapist encouraged the health visitor to use the work manual developed for children with hyperactivity[24] and to focus on clear messages and eye contact, making sure the child was listening. She encouraged the health visitor to discuss with the mother the background to why a child may be overactive, explaining that she might want to adapt her parenting style to a child with this particular difficulty. It was suggested that the health visitor visit the playgroup to discuss with the staff ways of handling the child.

Gradually Mrs Smith was able to feel more successful in managing her child and began to have more fun with her. The health visitor agreed with the mother that she would track the child through until school and discuss with the school nurse the possibility that this child might have some difficulty in school. This meant that, should the child's difficulties not settle gradually, she could be referred to the clinic for further assessment and treatment.

Work with school nurses

The Priestlands Pyramid Project was set up based on primary prevention principles[25] and is similar to the work of Appleton and colleagues in the Flintshire Project.[26] Over four years we worked with the headmasters of 10 primary schools that fed into one secondary school in the New Forest. The headmasters were concerned that many children in their schools had difficult behaviour and they realised that the different agencies did not have the capacity to deal with them.[27,28] They wanted SCAMHS, educational welfare officers, educational psychologists, and social services to work more closely together to prevent duplication of resources, and for the agencies to support the school. A joint protocol was drawn up.

A research project was started in order to evaluate the work. Several different projects were developed under the supervision of a project team consisting of representatives of the leaders, a consultant child psychiatrist, and senior staff from education and social services. A referral team was set up with a school nurse who liaised with the SCAMHS, educational psychologist, educational welfare officer, and a social worker. A "one-stop referral meeting" took place, with all referrals coming from the schools channelled through this meeting (with permission of the family), and then a decision made as to the best person or agency to take up the referral. Joint assessments took place with the school nurse and the education welfare officer, and the objective was to avoid formal referrals to a tier three service. As the school nurse worked part of the week in the SCAMHS as a liaison school nurse and was well supported by one of the senior nurse therapists and the consultant child psychiatrist, she was able to decide whether a formal referral was needed. No psychiatric file was opened unless a child was formally referred into the SCAMHS. This work was supported by standards funding from the Department of Education and by the different agencies, freeing up session time for staff.

Case example: an emotionally disturbed 10 year old

One of the primary schools was concerned about a child aged 10 who seemed sad and unhappy. She sat at the back of the class, not taking part in lessons, and had stopped producing the work that she had done well. She began to stop attending school. After discussion of concerns with the school nurse, her teacher talked to the child's parents and received permission to refer her formally to the school nurse. After a visit to the family by the school nurse and educational welfare colleague, it became clear that there were marital difficulties that had escalated over the preceding year, and the parents were considering separating. Jane, the eldest child in the family, was upset about this and protective of her mother because there had been some family violence. She was concerned also about her younger brother and sister who attended the same primary school. It was agreed that the educational welfare officer would work closely with the mother and father to help them resolve their decisions and to attempt to involve the children appropriately in the discussions. The school nurse agreed with Jane to meet weekly at school for 20 minutes for support and to give her ideas as to how she could cope. It was made clear to Jane that her parents were happy with her talking to the school nurse and that she would not be seen as disloyal. Gradually, over the three months that the school nurse was involved, Jane became happier. Her parents decided to separate but talked it through with the children and explained that the father would keep in contact, although the children would live with their mother.

An antibullying package in school

Another part of the project was a bullying package formulated by the SCAMHS using cognitive principles. There was a three-day training period. The package was delivered by teachers and another therapist (school nurse, health visitor, or educational welfare officer) in a classroom setting for one hour a week for five weeks; teachers complemented the package with "circle time" each week. Through this package, the children were encouraged to think of their own and each other's needs, to think about feelings, and to begin to find skills to solve problems without resorting to aggression. This package worked well and was enjoyed by both teachers and children. Each school adapted it in different ways to suit their own particular needs. One school made it a whole school policy and began to prioritise the support of children who might be unhappy. Schools set up mentors – older children to provide support for the younger children. In parallel, the Hampshire Education Department invested in a playground programme that helped schools to put together lunchtime activities for the children with a trained supervising teacher, in order that the children would not be bored. This, as we know from other research, can help to reduce bullying.[28]

We used as a screening tool the *My Life at School* booklet.[29] The children were pleased to have an opportunity to discuss being bullied. The major problems were those of emotional bullying, especially by girls. It was clear from this research that boys were less likely to take responsibility for their actions and were less likely to appreciate other children's emotions. The bullying package seemed to help children to focus more clearly on these deficits. Boys who were seen by teachers to be hyperactive or to have conduct disorders were more likely to be bullied, whereas girls with good pro-social skills were less likely to be bullied.[30]

The "Sure Start" programme

Through the Sure Start initiative, the government has started to try to tackle the roots of children's behaviour problems. Money has been released for projects in areas of deprivation, targeting small communities of preschool children. Each project has been allowed to develop to suit the needs of that community, but all are expected to collect good baseline information and to meet national targets. For example, all families are to be visited by a health visitor and mothers are to be offered good community midwife care in order to improve the welfare of the baby and reduce obstetric complications.

There are good opportunities for SCAMHS to work alongside their community colleagues to target families for more intensive work and in training Sure Start workers. Because funds will be time limited, it is important to help establish systems that will enable a consistency in approach for the future. As Southampton City will become one of the pilot "City Sure Starts", and we also have one of the pilot "Rural Sure Starts" in the New Forest, we have been discussing how best to support the initiative; joint posts between SCAMHS and Sure Start could be a way forward, as has happened in other parts of the country.

It will be important to follow these children into the future to track long term outcomes. Academic departments of child and adolescent psychiatry have a place locally in supporting this task.

The work of the primary mental health worker

SCAMHS around the country have been considering how to support primary care colleagues, and many have recently developed a specialised role for a primary mental health worker to work more closely with the community. A PMHW may work in the community reasonably independently of other SCAMHS colleagues. They may work on a variety of tasks. It is a role well developed by the adult services and is usually performed by community psychiatric nurses.

A survey of the roles of the PMHW was sent to 169 English mental health trusts. There were 98 returns (59%), which indicated that 22 SCAMHS had established this role and a further 42 were planning this in the future. The PMHWs were spending about 35% of their time in primary care, offering consultation and training to primary health care workers, rather than direct work with families and children.[31] This could be a matter of debate. When Portsmouth District first developed PMHWs (following closure of inpatient units), the nurses were offering mainly consultation and training, and this made no difference to the waiting list. The PMHWs also had a separate management system and were not part of SCAMHS (Stevenson, personal communication). The service has subsequently changed to take referrals of families from their primary health colleagues with active caseloads, and the management is now integrated into the SCAMHS. The waiting list for the SCAMHS is going down.

Johnson,[32] with the backing of a steering group, set up a project in Yorkshire comparing the work in two districts with and without a PMHW. He found that the referrals to the specialist CAMH services went down in the district with the PMHW. His recipe for success for a PMHW is that the worker be a skilled mental health professional who is respected by the other agencies. He suggested that the work should be a mixture of training primary health workers, support and consultation, joint working when appropriate, and referral to SCAMHS when necessary. These referrals to SCAMHS should have a high priority so that they are dealt with quickly. No referral from the community should bypass the PMHW. Management should come from within the SCAMHS.

The advantages of PMHWs working in the community include easy accessibility and scope for early preventive work before problems become entrenched. The service can be accessible to families in their own areas, without the stigma of attendance at a psychiatric clinic. However, if the assessment or treatment plan requires more intensive intervention or involvement by more staff, then easy access to SCAMHS can occur.

Benson *et al.* (unpublished data) described a new 0–16 year team operating mainly at tier two, offering interventions to a locality. They offer training to primary health workers, up to eight sessions with families in the community, and joint working with primary health workers. The team filter more complex chronic and persistent problems to the tier three/four team. Their outcome measure was *Health of the Nation* Outcome Scales for Children and Adolescents.[33,34] There were good outcomes on a case by case basis and positive feedback from families. There was an increase in referrals to the tier two SCAMHS team from 82 to 257.

Leicester SCAMHS (2001; personal communication), through a series of surveys of primary care staff, have set up training programmes for primary care staff, social workers and others, and now offer an MSc for primary health care staff to enable focused skills training for work with children and adolescents with behaviour problems.

There is a network for PMHWs with 50 members.[35] Three conferences have been held to date (Network National Committee).[35]

Constraints on these new ways of working in primary care

All SCAMHS are overstretched and underresourced, and have had to redefine referral criteria. Most are overburdened with children with chronically complex problems, especially those with attention deficit/hyperactivity disorder (ADHD), which take up a lot of medical resources (62% of the author's case load are medicated children, usually those with ADHD). Patients in SCAMHS used to be seen an average of four times.[36,37] The most recent figures for our clinic indicate that the mean number of appointments patients kept in 1999 was seven, with increased number of appointments for those having psychotherapy and those on stimulant medication. Many clinics are moving toward multiagency referral protocols, and this means that more emphasis may be placed on work with children who are in care.

The temptation is to try to divert back to the community children and families who appear to have less serious problems. This can only be practical if everyone is clear about what can be dealt with by professionals in the community and if, in turn, those professionals feel competent and fully supported in this task, and have the time to do it and the right to refer back to SCAMHS if the problem is beyond their competence.

Working in the community is exciting and more could be contained there. However, professionals who wish to involve their primary colleagues must be aware of the constraints under which they work. General practitioners have only seven minutes on average to spend with a patient and many have had no training in paediatrics or mental health, and so feel very unconfident in this area.

School teachers are under increasing pressure with government interdicts and new commands. Inclusion policies impose pressure on teachers and the rest of the class, as well as the disturbed children themselves. Teachers told us that it was the continual flow of paper commands from within their own school and the government that caused them stress. Difficult pupils added to this (Hayden et al., unpublished data).

Our work on the ADHD research project with health visitors indicated clearly the need to keep people to task so that they have quality control over the work they are doing, which encourages them to be very clear and focused. A major problem for health visitors is that they are generalists. Therefore, apart from having a large case load, they describe difficulty focusing on one task such as a child's overactivity when the family has other pressing problems they wish to discuss, such as housing or marital difficulties.

Evidence base

A recent systematic review of treatment of child and adolescent mental health problems in primary care outlined the evidence for effectiveness of interventions in the primary care setting by both primary care staff and specialist staff working in primary care.[38] The efficacy of a consultation–liaison role between services and the evidence for efficacy for skills training packages for primary care staff were also reviewed. The report outlined some interesting and creative work but pointed out that, as yet, many of the interventions had not been subjected to rigorous evaluation and in none had cost effectiveness been evaluated. Few studies of intervention had shown change in professional practice or change at the level of the behaviour of the child or family.

However, there are now well evaluated parenting packages used in a variety of community settings that may be adapted for use and be amenable for evaluation in primary care settings. These include Webster-Stratton's group programmes,[39,40] the Fast Track project,[41] and other school based interventions.[42]

Future developments

A recent survey of work conducted at the interface of SCAMHS and primary care suggested that the majority were involved in training primary care workers, but only about one-third had a structured consultation service or established PMHW posts, whereas one-fifth were offering community clinics and joint case work.[43] There were more likely to be developments with primary care when the SCAMHS had established specialist teams for children with specific disorders or within certain age groups, and where they had a dedicated SCAMHS manager.

The paper concludes that, if development of work in primary care is to continue, then evaluation of the services, including cost effectiveness, will be important. Time spent away from SCAMHS core business (assessment and treatment of serious mental illness) will have to be weighed against time spent with primary care colleagues. Only two-thirds of the SCAMHS in that survey were in negotiation over resources with health purchasing authorities or primary care trusts, and only three had reached agreement.

Because primary care trusts will be commissioning most of the SCAMHS in the future, negotiation will need to take place with them to discuss priorities for resources and funding for new initiatives.

References

1   Meltzer H, Gatward R, Goodman R, Ford T. *Mental health of children and adolescents in Great Britain*. London: Office of National Statistics, HMSO, 2000.
2   Health Advisory Service. *Child psychiatry: the future*. London: Department of Health, 1995.
3   Kurtz Z. *Treating children well*. London: The Mental Health Foundation, 1996.
4   Audit Commission. *Children in mind: child and adolescent mental health services*. Portsmouth: Audit Commission, 1999.
5   National Health Service. *National service framework for mental health: modern standards and service models*. London: HMSO, 1999.
6   British Paediatric Association. *The future configuration of paediatric services*. London: British Paediatric Association, 1996.
7   Thompson MJJ, Bellenis C. A joint assessment and treatment service for the under fives. Work with the health visitor in a child guidance clinic – paper 1: method. *ACPP Newslett* 1992;**14**:221–7.
8   Hooper C, Thompson M. *Manual for professionals working with preschool children*. Southampton: Southampton Community Health Services Trust, 1997.
9   Hooper C, Thompson M. *Manual for professionals working with school age children*. Southampton: Southampton Community Health Services Trust, 1997.
10 Thompson M, Stevenson J, Sonuga-Barke EJS, *et al*. The mental health of preschool children and their mothers in a mixed urban/rural population 1. Prevalence and ecological factors. *Br J Psychiatry* 1996;**168**:16–20.
11 Richman N, Stevenson J, Graham P. *Preschool to school: a behaviour study*. London: Academic Press, 1982.
12 Thompson M, Polke L. *A randomised controlled trial of the treatment of sleep disorders in 2 to 4 year olds*. Poster presentation to the European Association of Child Psychiatrists, 1992.

13 Polke L, Thompson M. *The crying child*. Southampton: Southampton University Hospitals Community Unit, 1994.
14 Polke L, Thompson M. *Temper tantrums*. Southampton: Southampton University Hospitals Community Unit, 1994.
15 Polke L, Thompson M. *Sleep and settling in the first year*. Southampton: Southampton University Hospitals Community Unit, 1994.
16 Polke L, Thompson M. *Overactive children*. Southampton: Southampton University Hospitals Community Unit, 1994.
17 Polke L, Thompson M. *Sleeping problems*. Southampton: Southampton University Hospitals Community Unit, 1994.
18 Bellenis C, Thompson MJJ. A joint assessment and treatment service for the under fives: work with the health visitors in a child guidance clinic – paper 2: work done and outcome. *ACPP Newslett* 1992;**14**:262–6.
19 Sonuga-Barke EJS, Daley D, Thompson M, Laver-Bradbury C, Weeks C. Parent based therapies for preschool attention-deficit/hyperactivity disorder: a randomised controlled trial with a community sample. *J Am Acad Child Adolesc Psychiatry* 2001;**40**:402–8.
20 Sonuga-Barke EJS, Thompson M, Daley D, Laver-Bradbury C. Parent training for preschool attention deficit/hyperactivity disorder: is it effective as part of routine primary care? *J Consult Clin Psychol* 2002 (in press).
21 Thompson MJJ, Coll X, Wilkinson S, Uitenbroek D, Tobias A. Evaluation of a mental health service for young children: development, outcome and satisfaction. *Child Adolesc Mental Health* 2003;**8**:68–77
22 Routh D. Hyperactivity. In: Magreb P, ed. *Psychological management of paediatric problems*. Baltimore: University Press, 1978.
23 Buss AR, Plomin R. *Temperament: early developing personality traits*. Hillsdale, NJ: Lawrence Erlbaum, 1984.
24 Weeks A, Laver-Bradbury C, Thompson M. *Manual for professionals working with hyperactive children*. Southampton: Southampton Community Health Services Trust, 1999.
25 Caplan G. *Principles of preventative psychiatry*. London: Tavistock Press, 1964.
26 Appleton P, Hammond-Rowley S. Addressing the burden of child and adolescent mental health problems: a primary care model. *Child Psychol Psychiatry Rev* 2000;**5**: 9–16.
27 Thompson M. *The Priestland Project*. Presentation to Royal College of Psychiatrists, Faculty of Child and Adolescent Psychiatrists Residential Meeting, 2000.
28 Thompson M, Kermode A, Parsons H. *Bullying package: the Priestland Project*. Presentation to Royal College of Psychiatrists, Faculty of Child and Adolescent Psychiatrists Residential Meeting, 2000.
29 Sharp P, Arora T, Smith PK, Whitney I. How to measure bullying in your school. In: Sharp S, Smith PK, eds. *Tackling bullying in your school: a practical handbook for teachers*. London: Routledge, 1994.
30 Johnson HR, Thompson MJJ, Wilkinson S, Walsh L, Balding J, Wright V. Vulnerability to bullying: teacher reported conduct and emotional problems, hyperactivity, peer relationships, difficulties and prosocial behaviour in primary school children. *Educ Psychol* 2002;**22**(5):553–6.
31 Lacey I. The role of the primary health worker. *J Adv Nursing* 1999;**30**:220–8.
32 Johnson P. *Primary mental health link worker*. Presentation to Royal College of Psychiatrists, Faculty of Child and Adolescent Psychiatrists Residential Meeting, 2001.
33 Gowers SG, Harrington RC, Whitton A, *et al.* Brief scale for measuring the outcomes of emotional and behavioural disorders in children. Health of the Nation Outcome Scales for Children and Adolescents (HoNOSCA). *Br J Psychiatry* 1999;**174**:413–6.
34 Gowers SG, Harrington RC, Whitton A, *et al.* Health of the Nation Outcome Scales for Children and Adolescents (HoNOSCA). Glossary for HoNOSCA score sheet. *Br J Psychiatry* 1999;**174**:428–31.
35 http://groups.yahoo.com/group/pmhw/
36 Thompson M, Parry G. A comparative audit of referrals to a child guidance clinic, 1981–1987. *Assoc Child Psychol Psychiatry Newslett* 1991;**13**:15–23.
37 Hoare P, Norton B, Chisholm D, Parry-Jones W. An audit of seven thousand successive child and adolescent psychiatric referrals in Scotland. *Clin Child Psychol Psychiatry* 1996;**1**:229–49.

38   Bower P, Garralda E, Kramer T, Harrington R, Sibbald B. The treatment of child and adolescent mental health problems in primary care: a systematic review. *Fam Pract* 2001;**18**:373–82.
39   Webster-Stratton C, Kolpacaff M, Hollinsworth T. Self-administered video tape therapy for families with conduct-problem children. Comparison with two cost-effective treatments and a control group change. *J Consult Clin Psychol* 1988;**56**:558–66.
40   Scott S, Spender Q, Doolan M, Jacobs B, Aspland H. Mutlicentre controlled trial of parenting groups for childhood antisocial behaviour in clinical behaviour in clinical practice. *BMJ* 2001;**323**:194–8.
41   Conduct Problems Research Group. Initial impact of the Fast Track prevention trial for conduct problems: II. Classroom effects. *J Consult Clin Psychol* 1999;**67**:648–57.
42   Wells J, Barlow J, Stewart-Brown S. *A systemic review of universal approaches to mental health promotion in schools*. Oxford: University of Oxford, 2001.
43   Bradley S, Kramer T, Garralda ME, Bower P, Macdonald W, Sibbald B. Child and adolescent mental health interface work with primary services: a survey of NHS provider trusts. *Child and Adolescent Mental Health* (in press).

12: Working with paediatrics

GILLIAN C FORREST

Overview

Chronic physical illness carries an increased risk for maladjustment for the child and family.

Adjustment is related to many factors in the child and his or her environment, not just to the specific disease.

Liaison child psychiatry services can provide a variety of useful interventions including:

diagnosis and treatment of psychiatric disorders

consultation and support for paediatric teams

teaching and training on psychological aspects of illness in childhood

contributing to research.

Multidisciplinary and multiagency work is vital for the comprehensive care of sick children.

Introduction

Paediatric care tends to focus on promoting the physical and developmental wellbeing of children, and most paediatricians work in hospital settings and have received little training in the psychological aspects of illness. Conversely, many child psychiatrists and their teams concentrate on the psychological care of physically healthy children and their families, work in community clinics, and have little experience of physically ill or disabled children.

In order to improve the services we provide for ill children and their families, we must develop a greater understanding of their psychological needs and of the ways in which child psychiatric and paediatric teams can work together to provide more holistic and "joined up" services. This area of work is known as "liaison child psychiatry", or "child liaison consultation", and is becoming increasingly important as the care of seriously ill children becomes ever more technologically complex and emotionally demanding for the children, their families, and their clinical teams.[1,2]

Box 12.1 Psychological problems in paediatrics

Chronic illness and disability
Somatising disorders
Acute stress in children
Deliberate self harm.

Psychological problems in paediatrics

Chronic illness and disability

For over 30 years it has been recognised that chronically ill children are at greater risk for psychological problems than are healthy children. The Isle of Wight study[3] showed that this risk was approximately double, and a similar finding was reported in the Ontario Child Health Study.[4] Overall, around 20% of chronically ill children have psychological difficulties or maladjustment to their illness, which is twice the rate in the normal population.[5] This maladjustment takes many forms, such as the following: needle phobias, anticipatory nausea and vomiting; non-compliance with treatment or diet; school avoidance; social withdrawal; and relationship difficulties. Some children meet the criteria for psychiatric disorders (mainly emotional or conduct disorders), which can predate their physical illness or develop during its course.

Originally, it was thought that the cause of this vulnerability was specific to the disease itself. However, from recent reviews of the literature, it appears that this only holds true for brain diseases. For other conditions, a child's adjustment is determined by the interplay between the disease, and risk and protective factors in the child, the family, and the environment (Figure 12.1).[6-8] These factors include the following:

- the child's developmental stage, temperament, and coping style prior to the illness
- the disease itself, its treatment (including hospitalisation), and the perception of its severity
- parental attitudes, family cohesion, and stability
- in the environment, the attitudes of the care team, the child's peer group, and school.

Lask[9] termed this "the illness network". In general, psychological disturbance is more likely to occur when these factors occur together. For example, psychological problems may develop in a younger child, with pre-existing psychological difficulties, with a chronic illness needing multiple hospitalisations, whose parents have an inappropriate

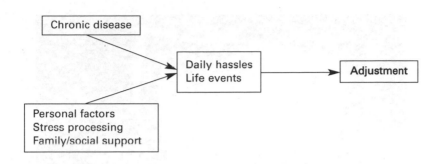

Figure 12.1 Adjustment

understanding of and reaction to the illness, and where the parent–child relationship is poor.[10]

Those involved in the care of a chronically ill child must be able to assess all of these factors in order to gain a full understanding of the child's predicament and to aid decision making about optimal care for the individual child and family. They must also be aware that a child's adjustment may fluctuate over time, with changes such as new life events increasing vulnerability, or improved coping skills with increased maturity decreasing the risk.

The care plan may need to include psychological therapy for the ill child, a parent or sibling; work with the whole family; or work with the network of professionals who are involved in the child's care (the paediatric team, the primary care team, and the teachers, among others). Skills beyond those that are available in the paediatric team are often needed, and here a close working relationship with a child psychiatry team can enable such comprehensive assessment and care to take place.

Somatising disorders

There are some chronic disabling illnesses for which no organic pathology can be demonstrated. Around one-third of children attending their primary care physician are found to be suffering from conditions in which psychological, rather than physical, factors are playing a major role in their ill health,[11,12] for example disorders of gait, headaches, and abdominal pain without any demonstrable organic cause. Most of these children are managed well by their parents and doctors, who recognise that worries about home or school can cause such symptoms, and help the child with reassurance and identifying the cause of the distress. However, there are some children whose symptoms, such as chronic fatigue or pain, are more severe, persistent or disabling, and whose parents continue to seek a physical explanation in spite of negative test results. In a few cases,

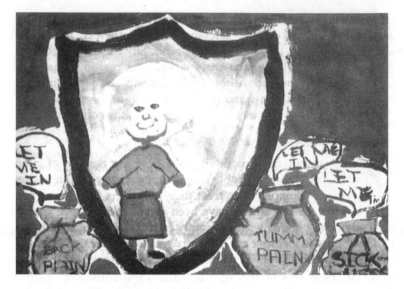

Stress can be manifested by pain in children

the child's physical symptoms such as skin lesions, seizures, or haematuria have been intentionally produced or feigned by the child or the parents (factitious illness).[13]

Children with these "somatising disorders" often fail to improve with routine paediatric care, and may get worse with continuing physical investigation. Here too, paediatricians and psychiatrists need to work closely together in order to enable an accurate diagnosis to be made and appropriate treatment plans put in place.[14,15]

Acute stress and children

Children with serious physical injuries can experience acute stress reactions alongside their injuries. This is particularly common with severe burns and after road traffic accidents, but can also be seen after traumatic procedures (such as painful injections or enemas) and physical or sexual abuse. Sometimes, these children have also had to cope with the death or injury of other members of their family in the same incident, as is frequently the case after major disasters. Relatives and paediatric staff are often overwhelmed by the distress experienced by these children, and psychological support and guidance may be helpful in preventing longer term post-traumatic stress reactions.[16] In post-traumatic stress disorder, children experience chronically high levels of anxiety and arousal, repeated re-experiencing of the trauma as flashbacks or bad dreams, and avoidance of any situations that would remind them of the trauma. In the early stages, supporting family cohesion, providing clear and accurate information about what happened, and encouraging the open expression of feelings directly or through play is generally recommended.[17,18] Specific cognitive behavioural approaches for anxiety or insomnia may be needed later.

Deliberate self harm

Deliberate self harm rises to a peak incidence in those aged 15–29 years, although it does occur under the age of 12.[19] Most children who self harm are reacting impulsively to conflicts within their relationships at home or with their peer group, and most are not seriously depressed. An acute stress such as sexual or physical abuse may be the precipitant, but in many cases the child has been made vulnerable to feelings of anger or rejection by a multiplicity of prior and current adversities in their family backgrounds and at school.[20] Of children and young people who self harm, 20% have made a previous attempt, and the risk for suicide must always be assessed by a mental health professional. Background factors must be identified, any psychiatric condition diagnosed, and appropriate care plans made. This may involve crisis intervention with the family, ongoing outpatient work, or even admission to a psychiatric ward.[21]

Working with paediatrics: the liaison child psychiatry model

The key to an effective psychosocial service for ill children, their families, and staff is an integrated approach between the paediatric and psychiatric teams.[22] There are many different models for achieving this, but however the services are organised they share certain characteristics that differentiate them from adult liaison services. A developmental and family systems perspective is needed for working with ill children; the emotional reactions of staff to ill and dying children are more intense; and the possible traumatic effects of hospitalisation and the need for special therapeutic techniques for hospitalised children must be taken into account.[22]

In general, the child psychiatrist working alone in a hospital setting has now largely been superseded by the multidisciplinary psychosocial team, working with children in hospital and outpatient clinic settings. This team may include child psychiatrists, child psychiatric nurses, clinical psychologists, specialist social workers, and therapists, who can offer a range of assessments and individual and family interventions, including non-verbal therapies (using art or play) for younger children.

The specific characteristics of any service are related both to the paediatric service (for example, oncology, nephrology, general paediatric or intensive care wards, community clinics) and to the psychological/psychiatric resources available, including whether staff are full members of the paediatric team or consult only.[23-25]

Most services are built around achieving good liaison and communication through psychosocial ward rounds or meetings. In this setting, paediatric and child psychiatry teams meet, and case centred discussions, staff support, and skills development through teaching can take place. The psychosocial meeting can also provide a valuable forum for developing a better understanding of the different attitudes and approaches of paediatricians and child psychiatrists toward psychological issues, and a forum in which tensions and disagreements between professionals can be aired and worked through.[9]

The main functions of a liaison child psychiatry service are summarised in Box 12.2.

Box 12.2 Main functions of a liaison child psychiatry service

Consultation and support for paediatric teams
Diagnosis and treatment of psychiatric disorders
Help with alleviating psychological issues (including major family problems) that are impeding the child's response to treatment
Sharing the care of complex chronic conditions, for example central nervous system disorders
Help with the management of acute stress reactions in traumatised children
Psychological care and advice for dying/bereaved children, their families, and the staff
Teaching and training on psychological aspects of illness in childhood
Contributing to research.

Using liaison child psychiatry services: case examples

Staff support: two girls with malignancies

Case example 1

Sara developed leukaemia when she was aged 10. Her parents had divorced several years earlier, and she lived with her mother, visiting her father regularly at weekends and holidays. Sara accepted her illness and treatment without major psychological upset, as did her father. Her mother, however, reacted with a mixture of anger and anxiety, and was extremely demanding of the doctors' and nurses' time on the ward. As time went by, and reassurance and information failed to help Sara's mother's stress, the staff started to feel increasingly helpless and frustrated, and began to be more openly critical of her. They felt that her behaviour was having a negative impact on Sara, who looked pained and sad whenever she witnessed her mother criticising the staff. They started to avoid the mother as much as possible, which in turn increased the mother's critical and demanding behaviour. The ward staff brought this to the weekly psychosocial ward round, which was attended by the paediatric consultant and junior doctors, nursing staff, play specialists, dietician, and the hospital social worker. After a full discussion of the psychological issues in the family and the feelings of the staff concerned, they were able to adopt a more supportive attitude toward Sara's mother. As a result, the situation eased.

Case example 2

A 14 year old girl needed an amputation because of a malignant bone tumour. Her mother was terrified of the girl's reaction to this news, and begged the surgeon not to tell her until the last moment before the operation. The surgeon too was finding this situation very stressful, and was inclined to follow the mother's wishes. However, after discussing the issues with the child psychiatrist, the hospital social worker, and the ward staff at the psychosocial meeting, he realised that the girl needed to be given time to accept the necessity for this mutilating surgery, and to have support for the intense emotional reaction that would accompany it.

Discussion

These cases illustrate the way in which consultation with the psychosocial team can improve quality of care by addressing the emotional impact on staff of a child's illness. By providing space for the staff to explore and communicate their reactions, ways can be found to help them cope effectively with the wide range of emotionally demanding situations that occur in paediatric care.[26-28]

Maladjustment in chronic illness: a girl with diabetes

Mary, at age six, had had diabetes for two years. She coped quite well initially, until her father also developed the disease a year later. From then on, Mary became oppositional about all aspects of her treatment, refusing her diet, screaming when her insulin injections were given, and generally being uncooperative and angry at home, with frequent fights with her younger brother and tantrums over minor frustrations. Both her paediatrician and her parents were extremely worried about her diabetic control, and referred her to the child liaison team.

After discussions with the diabetic community nurse, who knew the family well, they were offered a series of meetings in the child psychiatry clinic. It quickly became clear that Mary's mother was significantly depressed. Her father was having great difficulties coming to terms with his own condition, and was so preoccupied with it that he had withdrawn from any aspect of Mary's diabetic care, leaving her mother unsupported. She in turn was grieving the loss of normal family life, and of her role as effective guardian and protector of her child. As a consequence, she had lost her capacity to set firm limits and boundaries. Mary's brother was resentful that all the available parental attention in the family was now focused on Mary, and lost no opportunity to pick quarrels with her to act out his anger.

The parents had some sessions alone to explore the impact of the father's illness on their relationship, and were able to talk for the first time about their reaction to the father becoming diabetic. Mother was persuaded to consult her general practitioner about her depression and she was prescribed a course of antidepressants. A joint plan was made with the diabetic community nurse to support mother in limit setting for Mary, with a reward system (star chart) for compliance with injections and diet. Mary's brother was included in several meetings exploring the conflict between the children, and plans were agreed for him to have some special time set aside for him by each parent.

Mary's parents' relationship improved steadily, and alongside this Mary's behaviour improved too and the fighting between the siblings stopped. Within three months she was again fully cooperating with her treatment.

Discussion

There is much literature on the psychological aspects of diabetes, and there is some evidence that individual analytical therapy, family therapy, and behaviour therapy can all be helpful.[2] Like most diabetic children, however, Mary adjusted well initially to her illness.[29] It was the additional stress of her father's illness that overwhelmed the family's coping strategies and precipitated serious emotional and behaviour problems in the family. Therapy for all of the family members was necessary to alleviate Mary's oppositional defiant disorder.

Parental maladjustment is related to child maladjustment in chronic illness, and may need attention in its own right or as part of family work. The needs of siblings of chronically ill and disabled children are often overlooked, and this can result in lowered self esteem, depression, and social isolation.[30,31] Finding ways to help stressed parents to share the available attention between their children without increasing any feelings of guilt requires sensitivity and skill.

The case also illustrates the importance of linking with other parts of the "illness network", in this case the general practitioner and the diabetic nurse.

Psychological problems impeding treatment and self concept in chronic illness: a girl with immune deficiency syndrome

Anne was the only child of loving parents. She was born with common variable immune deficiency syndrome and survived until her 28th year. She was a happy and popular girl at primary school, in spite of many episodes of illness, including respiratory infections, nephritis, and uveitis. The family coped well with her father's treatment for cancer when she was five years old. At eight years she developed severe bronchiectasis and was offered an experimental new treatment – a course of painful intramuscular injections. Her parents became very anxious about her prognosis, and Anne developed a needle phobia and was completely resistant to treatment. She became very depressed and her play became dominated by themes of death and dying.

She was referred to the child liaison team for psychological help, and after close discussions with her parents and the paediatric team she was offered a combination of art therapy, which she used to communicate her fears of dying, and behavioural treatment of her needle phobia. She improved steadily and was able to complete the course of injections successfully.

Discussion

Anne had a chronic progressive condition but was well adjusted until her disease reached a critical point when she was eight. Protective factors in her case were her good temperament, stable family background, and the supportive environment provided by the paediatric team and at school. She became vulnerable when she became able to appraise the life threatening nature of her condition. This process of changing self concept in chronic illness is linked both to the child's developmental stage and understanding of death,[32,33] and with their own experience of the life threatening nature of their illness, as judged by, for example, a relapse or knowledge of the death of other affected children or adults.[34] Anne recognised the seriousness of her condition through the reactions of her parents and doctors to her deteriorating lung function, and her referral for an experimental new drug trial.

With psychological help, however, she was able to form new coping strategies for containing her anxieties about dying, and so was able to continue accepting active treatment for her condition.

Somatising disorder: a boy with limb and abdominal pains

Alan aged 10 was a bright child with a perfectionist temperament. He had been investigated for gastrointestinal problems by a hospital specialist when he was seven, with inconclusive results. A grandparent had died of cancer the year before his illness developed.

He presented with a three-month history of pains in his limbs and abdomen. Extensive investigations were all negative, and additional symptoms appeared – photophobia, headache, and difficulty walking. He was admitted to a paediatric ward for further tests, which were again negative, but he deteriorated and started refusing solid food. He was highly anxious and depressed, and unable to cope with washing, dressing, or feeding himself. His mother was convinced that he had an undiagnosed malignant disease.

With the combined input of the paediatrician and child psychiatrist, his parents were eventually persuaded to try a psychological approach to his treatment. He was transferred to a child psychiatric unit as a day patient, and individual therapy and family work was started, along with physiotherapy and a behavioural programme aimed at managing his pain and increasing his self confidence. As his parents became more robust and confident of his recovery, Alan became more able to verbalise his angry feelings related to the death of his grandfather, his sibling rivalry, and his problems with his peer relationships at school. After help for him and his family with these difficulties, his physical symptoms gradually improved. He eventually made a full recovery and returned to school, with close liaison between his teachers and the psychiatric team.

Discussion

Alan had a somatoform disorder, and shared many of the typical features of such children. He had a perfectionist temperament with anxiety traits and low self esteem; in his family there was an anxious preoccupation with illness, and his grandparent provided the model for his symptoms.[15,35] Stress in the school environment (in Alan's case his difficult relationships with his peer group) is often also a factor. In about one-third of the children, co-morbid emotional disorder (depression or anxiety disorder) is present, often developing during the course of the illness. Finding a way to engage the child and family in addressing the underpinning psychological factors is frequently challenging for the paediatrician and child psychiatrist. Once the correct diagnosis was reached, and Alan's parents engaged, investigations could be halted and attention focused on the psychological issues. Alan's physical symptoms had been serving to express his inner pain. He needed help to start to put these feelings into words. Like many of the children, however, he also needed a programme of graded rehabilitation drawn up by a physiotherapist and occupational therapist, and his pain needed a careful programme of behaviour management, alongside ongoing family work.[14] His return to school required careful liaison with the education department.

Joint care of a complex disorder: a boy with severe generalised epilepsy

Michael was referred by his paediatrician at age seven years. He had severe generalised epilepsy from age three, which was treated with anticonvulsants. Since starting school at five, his behaviour had become increasingly difficult at home and school, with poor concentration, overactivity, mood swings, and violent outbursts when thwarted. He was the older of two children. His father was a strict disciplinarian, and his mother worked as a health care assistant and had a more tolerant and permissive parenting style.

Michael was assessed by the liaison team and met the diagnostic criteria for hyperkinetic disorder (attention deficit/hyperactivity disorder) and specific learning difficulties. His treatment was complicated both by his seizure disorder and the inconsistencies in management by his parents and teachers. Joint work with the child psychiatrist and paediatrician enabled an appropriate medication regimen to be achieved. Parent counselling by the team's social worker helped to improve parental consistency. Liaison with the school helped them to understand and manage Michael's learning difficulties and problem behaviour in that setting more effectively. Ongoing joint work has been necessary to manage a severe episode of maternal depression, the development of a tic disorder, and sibling rivalry, which culminated at one point in Michael's brother refusing school. Michael's seizure control remains less than perfect, and his move to secondary school presents a new set of challenges.

Discussion

Brain disorders and epilepsy carry heightened risks for psychiatric disorder and family difficulties.[3,36] The complexity of Michael's needs required the combined skills of the paediatric and psychosocial team, particularly over the use of medication.

Work with issues of seizure control, child and family adjustment, peer relationships, and special educational needs simultaneously is often necessary. Like all chronic conditions, vulnerabilities change over time, but the transition to secondary school is often a major event that requires much interprofessional and interagency collaboration.

Training and education

The psychosocial ward round, case presentations, and other joint meetings provide excellent opportunities for teaching and training on the psychosocial aspects of childhood illness, including the ethical issues surrounding the care of sick children, and staff stress. In addition, the team can contribute to the formal undergraduate and postgraduate training programmes. Techniques familiar to child mental health professionals, such as the use of videos and role play, are particularly well suited to this area of teaching.

Research

There is still a great deal to learn about the psychological aspects of illness and disability, and the outcomes of psychological interventions with ill children and their families. More attention needs to be paid to the role of fathers in particular, and to the effect of the child's social context (peer group, school, and treatment setting), and longitudinal studies are needed to examine the effects of chronic illnesses on child development.[8,37] The liaison child psychiatry team is well placed to contribute to studies in these areas, in collaboration with teams in other centres.

Contraindications

There are really no contraindications to involving the liaison child psychiatry team, provided any resistance to psychological assessment on the part of the child and family can be overcome first. There is still a widely held belief that a physical cause for illness is legitimate, but a psychological cause implies madness or malingering. The paediatrician may well have to approach these issues directly with parents, reassuring them about the interplay between physical and psychological factors in illness, and emphasising that psychosomatic symptoms are as real and disabling as symptoms with an organic cause.[15] It is often most helpful when the child psychiatrist (and team) can be introduced to vulnerable children and families at an early stage, as part of the team providing comprehensive care for the child and family.[9]

Implications for multiagency working

Successful holistic care of ill and disabled children needs to encompass every aspect of their lives. This will include their school and social environment, as well as the health care network of primary and specialist care. The hospital school and home tuition services play vital roles in maintaining the child's education while too ill for school, thus helping to normalise the child's life as much as possible, as well as providing occupation and opportunities to boost self esteem. Educational psychologists, special needs coordinators, and education officers may all be needed to set up integration programmes for children returning to school with special needs related to their condition. Close liaison with the paediatric and child psychiatry teams and pre-discharge planning will help to ensure that all aspects are known about and catered for.

Links with social services departments may be facilitated if there are social workers attached to the paediatric or liaison teams, so that any concerns about inadequate living conditions or child protection (abuse or neglect) can be addressed while the child is in hospital, and family support can be planned if necessary.[38] Occasionally, alternative placements may be needed for a child whose family can no longer provide care, and close links with foster families will be needed to help them to understand the child's physical and emotional needs and make appropriate plans.

For the child with a terminal condition for which palliative care is required, there may be a large network of statutory and voluntary agencies whose input needs to be coordinated. The paediatric and liaison child psychiatry services are well placed to undertake this role, together with the primary health care team, in order to plan for the needs of the child, family, and professionals.

Where a parent is suffering from a serious psychiatric disorder such as schizophrenia, or substance abuse, the liaison child psychiatrist will need to link with the adult psychiatric service to ensure that the child's needs are understood, alongside the needs of the ill parent. There will also be circumstances in which the liaison child psychiatrist identifies serious psychiatric problems in a parent, and liaises with adult psychiatric colleagues to agree and facilitate referral to an appropriate source of help.

Conclusion

Working with paediatrics to provide comprehensive care for ill children, their families, and staff is both challenging and rewarding. Services remain patchy and information about effective interventions is still at an early stage. Nevertheless, significant progress is being made, and as the need for better children's services moves higher up the agenda of providers and commissioners of health care, we can anticipate the development of more integrated and effective, better resourced services.

References

1 Knapp PK, Harris E. Consultation-liaison psychiatry: a review of the past 10 years. Part 1: clinical findings. *J Am Acad Child Adolesc Psychiatry* 1998;37:17–25.
2 Graham P, Turk J, Verhulst F. Psychosocial aspects of physical disorders: general. In: *Child psychiatry, a developmental approach*. Oxford: Oxford University Press, 1999.

3 Rutter M, Tizard J, Whitmore K. *A neuropsychiatric study in childhood*. London: Heinemann, 1970.
4 Cadman D, Boyle M, Szatmari P, Offord DR. Chronic illness, disability, and mental and social well-being: findings of the Ontario Child Health Study. *Pediatrics* 1987;**79**:805–13.
5 Lavigne JV, Faier-Routman J. Correlates of psychosocial adjustment to pediatric physical disorders: a meta-analytic review and comparison with existing models. *J Dev Behav Pediatr* 1993;**14**:117–23.
6 Eiser C. Psychological effects of chronic disease. *J Child Psychol Psychiatry* 1990;**31**:85–98.
7 Mrazek DA. Psychiatric aspects of somatic disease and disorders. In: Rutter M, Taylor E, Hersov L, eds. *Child and adolescent psychiatry; modern approaches*, 3rd edn. Oxford: Blackwell Science, 1994.
8 Wallender JL, Varni JW. Effects of chronic physical disorders on child and family adjustment. *J Child Psychol Psychiatry* 1998;**39**:29–46.
9 Lask B. Paediatric liaison work. In: Rutter M, Taylor E, Hersov L, eds. *Child and adolescent psychiatry; modern approaches*, 3rd edn. Oxford: Blackwell Science, 1994.
10 Ortiz P. General principles in child liaison consultation: a literature review. *Eur Child Adolesc Psychiatry* 1997;**6**:1–6.
11 Cundall D. Children and mothers at clinics: who is disturbed? *Arch Dis Child* 1987;**55**:555–61.
12 Garralda ME, Bailey D. Psychosomatic aspects of children's consultations in primary care. *Arch Psychiatr Neurol Sci* 1987;**236**:319–22.
13 Eminson DM, Postlethwaite RJ. *Munchausen syndrome by proxy abuse: a practical approach*. Oxford: Butterworth-Heinemann, 2000.
14 Eminson DM. Somatising in children and adolescents. 1. Clinical presentations and aetiological factors. *Adv Psychiatr Treat* 2001;**7**:266–74.
15 Garralda ME. Assessment and management of somatisiation in childhood and adolescence: a practical perspective. *J Child Psychol Psychiatry* 1999;**40**:1159–67.
16 Yule W. Post traumatic stress disorder. In: Rutter M, Taylor E, Hersov L, eds. *Child and adolescent psychiatry; modern approaches*, 3rd edn. Oxford: Blackwell Science, 1994.
17 Udwin O. Children's reactions to traumatic events. *J Child Psychol Psychiatry* 1993;**34**:115–27.
18 Dyregrov A. *Grief in children*. London: Jessica Kingsley Publications, 1994.
19 Hawton K, Fagg J. Deliberate self-poisoning and self-injury in adolescents. A study of characteristics and trends in Oxford 1976–89. *Br J Psychiatry* 1992;**161**:816–23.
20 Goodman R, Scott S. Suicide and deliberate self-harm. In: *Child psychiatry*. Oxford: Blackwell Science, 1997.
21 Shaffer D, Piacentini J. Suicide and attempted suicide. In: Rutter M, Taylor E, Hersov L, eds. *Child and adolescent psychiatry; modern approaches*, 3rd edn. Oxford: Blackwell Science, 1994.
22 Taylor DC. The components of sickness: disease, illness and predicaments. In: Apley J, Ounsted C, eds. *One child*. London: Spastics International Medical Publications, 1982.
23 McFadyen A, Broster G, Black D. The impact of a child psychiatry liaison service on patterns of referral. *Br J Psychiatry* 1991;**158**:93–6.
24 Leslie SA. Paediatric liaison. *Arch Dis Child* 1992;**67**:1046–9.
25 North C, Eminson M. A review of a psychiatry-nephrology liaison service. *Eur Child Adolesc Psychiatry* 1998;**7**:235–45.
26 Lansdown R, Goldman A. The psychosocial care of children with malignant disease *J Child Psychol Psychiatry* 1988;**29**:555–67.
27 Vachon MLS, Pakes E. Staff stress in the care of the critically ill and dying child. In: Wass H, Corr CA, eds. *Childhood and death*. New York: Hemisphere Publishing, 1984:151–82.
28 Woolley H, Stein A, Forrest GC, Baum JD. Staff stress and job satisfaction at a children's hospice. *Arch Dis Child* 1989;**64**:114–8.
29 Northam E, Anderson P, Adler R, Werther G, Warne G. Psychosocial and family functioning in children with insulin dependent diabetes at diagnosis and one year later. *J Pediatr Psychol* 1996;**21**:699–717.

30 Breslau N, Prabucki K. Siblings of disabled children. *Arch Gen Psychiatry* 1987;**44**:1040–6.
31 Drotar D, Crawford P. Psychological adaptation of siblings of chronically ill children: research and practice implications. *Dev Behav Pediatrics* 1985;6:355–62.
32 Kane B. Children's concepts of death. *J Genet Psychol* 1979;**134**:141–53.
33 Lansdown R, Benjamin G. The development of the concept of death in children aged 5 to 9 years. *Child Care Health Dev* 1985;**11**:13–20.
34 Bluebond Langner M. *The private lives of dying children*. Princeton, NJ: Princeton University Press, 1978.
35 Walker LS, Garber J, Greene JW. Somatic complaints in pediatric patients: a prospective study of the role of negative life events, child social and academic competence and parental somatic symptoms. *J Consult Clin Psychol* 1993;**62**: 1213–21.
36 Goodman R. Brain disorders. In: Rutter M, Taylor E, Hersov L, eds. *Child and adolescent psychiatry; modern approaches*, 3rd edn. Oxford: Blackwell Science, 1994.
37 Knapp PK, Harris E. Consultation-liaison psychiatry: a review of the past 10 years. Part 2: research on treatment approaches and outcomes *J Am Acad Child Adolesc Psychiatry* 1998;**37**:139–46.
38 Jones DPH, Byrne G, Newbould C. Management, treatment and outcomes. In: Eminson DM, Postlethwaite RJ, eds. *Munchausen syndrome by proxy abuse: a practical approach*. Oxford: Butterworth-Heinemann, 2000.

13: Working with education

BRIDGET O'SHEA

Overview

Child mental health practitioners and teachers should work closely together to manage problems causing distress for pupils.
Joint activities may include:
sharing knowledge on an individual child's difficulties
behavioural principles underpinning school and classroom management
liaison regarding the educational needs of children with learning difficulties or in other special circumstances such as refugees
treatment of particular problems causing an impact on school life, such as attention deficit/hyperactivity disorder or school refusal.

Introduction

Child and Adolescent Mental Health Services (CAMHS) have varying degrees of intensity of contact with educational services. In the UK, however, school attendance is mandatory from five until sixteen years of age. School life will therefore occupy a large proportion of a child's existence and will have a significant influence on successful development. For this reason child mental health professionals should have a vested interest in establishing strong links with their local education authority at all levels.

School factors

It has long been established that particular school qualities have an effect on pupil behaviour and achievement. CAMHS staff quickly learn which local schools have especially high rates of behavioural problems. The "15,000 hours" study (aptly named to reflect the number of hours of childhood spent in the school environment) clearly demonstrated differences between educational, social, and behavioural outcomes among schools within the same area, depending on the ethos of the school.[1] Appropriate social functioning and academic achievement is fostered in schools where there is a reinforcement of appropriate behaviour and an orderly environment.

There should be an emphasis on academic work, with teachers acting as strong role models, and sharing of roles and responsibilities so that subgroups of pupils do not become alienated. An effective behavioural policy that is clearly stated allows the early identification and management of any behavioural problems.

Variety of contact between Child and Adolescent Mental Health Services and school staff

The primary contact between schools and CAMHS staff will be regarding individual patients. The referral rate of children and adolescents to child mental health services by education professionals may differ considerably between services, as shown by Yates et al.[2] This is likely to reflect historical patterns of service development and an emphasis on different priorities in overly stretched services. In addition, there is a general trend toward increased recognition of particular conditions that have an important impact on children's school careers, such as attention deficit/hyperactivity disorder (ADHD). Current political agendas for social inclusion – the maintenance of disaffected pupils within a mainstream setting – may also have an impact on referral patterns and lead to an increase in requests for CAMHS involvement. Discussions about the diagnostic presentation of these referrals and response to various treatments can greatly aid therapeutic programmes; for example, the short half life of many stimulant medications used to treat ADHD necessitates their administration in school time.

Contact with education colleagues regarding pupils may be of a varied nature. A non-exhaustive list is outlined in Box 13.1.

Box 13.1 Contact between schools and Child and Adolescent Mental Health Services

Requests for school reports from class teachers to aid in diagnostic assessment.

Completion of questionnaires to aid diagnosis and for monitoring of treatment response.

Observation of children within the classroom by CAMHS professionals.

Preparation of reports to contribute to assessment of special educational needs.

Consultation work within specialist school settings, such as those for emotionally and behaviourally disturbed pupils.

Liaison with schools regarding particular conditions with a large classroom impact, such as ADHD and conduct disorders.

Outreach work by CAMHS professionals within schools with particularly vulnerable groups, such as refugees and asylum seekers.

Placement of teachers within CAMHS day units and inpatient units.

Information required from schools for Child and Adolescent Mental Health Service assessments

The initial contact between CAMHS and school staff will usually be in the form of a request for a report on the child before a diagnostic appointment. The importance of high quality informative data should not be underestimated. Next to parents, it is likely that no other care giver has spent more time with a child than a teacher. The school should only be approached to provide a report if there is prior permission from the child's parents. If the family's general practitioner makes the referral, then the parents can be made aware of the importance of this process. Permission to contact a school can be obtained in writing before the family's first appointment. It is usually assumed, if a referral is received from a head teacher or teacher with responsibility for special educational needs, that the parent has a full understanding of the school's concerns, but this is not always the case. Confusion can arise, particularly if there are different perspectives between the parents and the school in question. In some cases, symptoms may only be present in one setting. In these incidences it may be wise to have a meeting with all concerned to clarify the reasons for CAMHS involvement.

The information on how to access external resources for all pupils should be set out in a local education authority behaviour support plan.

Information from schools is essential in diagnostic assessments because children may behave differently in different settings. A more pervasive problem (i.e. one that presents itself both in home and school environments) is usually of greater significance. Information that is usefully obtained is outlined in Box 13.2.

Box 13.2 Helpful school information for child psychiatric assessments

The pupil's attendance record.
Behaviour in the classroom and the playground.
Any concern about their impulse control or activity levels.
Academic strengths and weaknesses, with particular attention to reading skills.
The pupil's social relationships with teachers and their peers.
Whether the child has received any school evaluation to obtain additional education resources.
Any other observations of importance.

It can be useful to explain to teachers providing reports that their information is immensely helpful but that detailed replies regarding the outcome of an assessment are not permissible because of issues of medical confidentiality.

Questionnaires

In addition to verbal or written reports, questionnaires can provide useful additional information for assessment and a baseline against which to measure the effectiveness of an intervention. However, they should not be seen as a substitute for personal discussion or a report from a teacher. One of the most user friendly questionnaires is Goodman's Strengths and Difficulties Questionnaire.[3] This is because of the presence of the pro-social subscale which, unlike many other scales, records positive responses. Other questionnaires used may include those for specific diagnoses such as ADHD, for which the Conners' Teachers Scale may be employed.[4]

Contributions to special educational needs assessment

The Warnock Report in 1989 established that as many as 20% of children may have some sort of learning difficulty that may require specialist provision at certain times in their school careers. This may range from extra teacher support within the classroom to placement within a specialist school (for example, for autism, a sensory handicap, emotional or behaviour problems, or learning disability). In cases of severe handicap it will be apparent from before school that a specialist education placement is necessary. Other children may be identified as having learning or behavioural problems after school entry.

The roles and responsibilities of professionals in relation to children with special educational needs are set out within a code of practice document.[5] Teachers are required to identify and assess any pupil who they consider to have special educational needs. A nominated teacher acts as a special education needs coordinator (SENCO) and takes particular responsibility for these children, and has a liaison role with external agencies. After an educational assessment has been carried out, teaching strategies and targets for the child are put in place and recorded in an individual education plan. This stage of intervention is termed "School Action", and input may range from extra one-to-one or group teaching support to the provision of special materials or learning equipment. If the child fails to make progress over a period of time, then the advice of an external specialist such as an educational psychologist or behaviour advisory teacher is sought under the intervention "School Action Plus". The aim of intervention is to deliver support within a mainstream setting. In a small number of cases further input is advisable, and the local education authority must undertake a full assessment that may lead to a statement of their special educational needs (Education Act, 1996). Information is gathered from parents, the class teacher and SENCO, educational

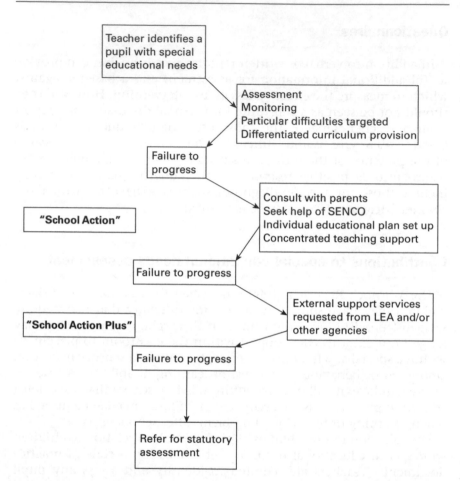

Figure 13.1 Pathway for assessment and monitoring of pupils with special educational needs who progress to statutory assessment. LEA, local education authority; SENCO, special education needs coordinator

psychologist, and any other professional involved with the child. Doctors and other professionals also have the right to request a statutory assessment in cases where they feel the child's educational needs are not being met. This process is summarised in Figure 13.1.

At any stage health professionals may be involved with the child in question and medical reports may be requested as a contribution to the assessment of special educational needs. Medical reports should address the physical and psychological needs of the child. It is not permissible to recommend a specific school within the report but guidance may be given on the type of environment and appropriate classroom strategies that may be useful. For example, a child or young person with ADHD would benefit from a low distractibility setting with frequent prompts to remain on task and brief academic assignments.

All reports are shown to parents together with the final statement. It is courteous to disclose the contents of the medical report to parents before submission. If there are any parental objections to medical or family details in the reports, then they should be omitted; statement contributions form part of the child's education record and are not therefore confidential. It is also worth noting that the overall time frame requires parents to receive written notification of the outcome of assessment within 12 weeks of a decision being made that an assessment should occur, and so reports should be submitted promptly.

Case example: behavioural problems secondary to learning difficulties

A 14 year old boy, A, was referred to CAMHS by his school SENCO. He had displayed loud, silly, and childish behaviour in class for over a year. He was rude and defiant to teachers, and on one occasion was excluded for attempting to tie a piece of tape around a teacher's neck. At home there was no oppositional or actively aggressive behaviour. He seemed uncommunicative and was possibly depressed.

A's early milestones were unremarkable apart from slow speech and language development. He received speech and language therapy at the age of three because he did not use sentences. Through his primary school years he received additional support for specific difficulties in communication but a request for statutory assessment of special educational need was rejected.

A's difficult classroom behaviour was initially tackled by a thorough assessment. His school requested an educational psychologist's opinion. This revealed that A had a marked performance and verbal IQ discrepancy. He had difficulties with all aspects of comprehension, and his expressive language abilities were the equivalent of those in a six year old.

The child psychiatry team were able to liaise with educational staff to establish that A's behaviour was secondary to his learning anomalies. It was apparent that, although A had learnt to read and write to an adequate level, he had no real grasp of the full use of these tasks. He had difficulties knowing how to behave in a busy classroom situation, and found movement around a large school confusing. His deterioration coincided with the increasing demands of the secondary school curriculum.

A was admitted to a CAMHS day unit but, in spite of the intensive support offered, his behaviour continued to deteriorate and he was permanently excluded from his mainstream school. The unit staff submitted reports to the special needs panel emphasising that his behaviour difficulties were secondary to his unaddressed learning difficulties. The statutory assessment of A's needs concluded that he would not benefit from transfer to a further mainstream school. Although the majority of children's special educational needs are met locally, A was eventually successfully integrated into a residential boarding school that also had the capacity to cater for his marked specific learning difficulty because there was no local school with this capability. His psychiatric symptoms had all resolved at this stage and his parents reported improved communication with him at home.

Disruption and overactivity

Working with education necessitates liaison with teachers over conditions that are extremely common and cause significant classroom impact. The bulk of referrals to CAMHS involve children with problems that cause significant disruption in their lives and the lives of those around them. Up to 50% have conduct disorders and a proportion of these will have co-morbid ADHD. The most common period for teachers to become concerned about their pupils' activity levels is during the early primary school years. As children progress through the education system there is an increasing expectation for them to sit still, concentrate, and complete work assignments. Once referred to CAMHS and in assessment, a very useful means of confirming a diagnosis is a classroom observation of a child while he or she performs an academic task.[6] Attention should be paid to the features of hyperactivity, time off task, inappropriate vocalisations, fidgetiness, and movement from the seat. If the teacher highlights an average class student, then this can be a useful comparison.

It is helpful to educate teachers about the causes and treatments of hyperactive behaviour. A combination of behavioural methods and stimulant medication produces the best results.[7] Strategies that may benefit a child with ADHD in the classroom include placing the child near to the teacher, reducing distractions, setting and maintaining limits, and the use of frequent positive comments to enhance self esteem. Clear and rapid systems of contingent reward and response cost promote compliant behaviour. Reading disability, which occurs with both conduct disorder and hyperactivity, can hamper educational progress. It is useful to screen for whether the child's reading age is significantly below that expected on the basis of chronological age and IQ.[8]

Children and young people with conduct and oppositional disorders frequently pose significant difficulties for overall classroom management. Aggressive children are more impulsive, have fewer problem solving skills, and have a tendency to attribute hostile intent to others in aggressive or ambiguous situations. McMahon[9] showed the efficacy of a primary preventive model targeting whole classrooms. Teachers can be trained to deliver social competence programmes that provide pupils with lessons on self control, emotional awareness, peer relations, and problem solving. Bullying situations can be reduced with curriculum based strategies that raise awareness of the feelings of victims, together with assertiveness training for the victims themselves. A drawback to the provision of these interventions is the requirement of considerable dedication and commitment from the schools concerned.

Specific guidelines are issued to schools regarding the management of truancy, bullying, and disruptive behaviour.[10] Particular strategies outlined include "circle of friends" (a peer remediation and support programme) and clear policies for unauthorised absence and for bullying. Pupils should be encouraged to report bullying incidents to staff that they can trust, or older pupils. School staff, including lunchtime supervisors, need to be alert to the signs of bullying and should act firmly, because the worst possible outcome of persistent and unrecognised bullying is suicide. Olweus[11] outlined a successful nationwide antibullying campaign undertaken in Norway.

School refusal

School refusal due to anxiety, in the absence of antisocial behaviour, is another common reason for referral to CAMHS by educational staff. Under the Education Act of 1996, a local education authority may prosecute parents if their child fails to attend school regularly. If the child is "ill", then prosecution can be deferred. Education welfare officers or education social workers work with schools and families to resolve attendance issues, and they are usually the key professional to aid in a school return programme. Blagg[12] gave a detailed account of assessment, diagnostic, and treatment issues. The main principle of management of school refusal should be to get the child back to school as quickly as possible using a behavioural approach. If there is access to a specialist unit in which teachers employed by the local education authority work with colleagues from a mental health setting, then this can provide intensive support.

Case example: school refusal

A 14 year old girl, C, had not attended school for a four-month period, after a three-year history of sporadic attendance. She had been anxious about going to school throughout her primary school years, and after secondary transfer she had had increasing amounts of time off school with tenuous illnesses. She had experienced some verbal taunting and rejection by her peer group but was reluctant to inform the school staff of the names of the individuals involved. She had changed school, with no resolution to her symptoms.

C was depressed, with prominent mood changes; she threatened to commit suicide if forced to go to school, but denied wishing this in any other context.

C's parents were very clear that they wished her to return to school. A meeting was held involving C and her parents, her education welfare officer, her school year head, and the CAMHS team. A school return programme was commenced, with behavioural reinforcement for each step of the programme that she completed successfully. She was coached in how to respond to questions from her peers about her absence and how to manage her anxiety through relaxation, distraction, and challenging her anxious thoughts.

The CAMHS team carefully planned C's reintegration back to school in order to ensure that the teaching staff were sympathetic to her. Her timetable was obtained and a visit to the school site undertaken to rehearse her reintegration with her year head. C's day unit teacher accompanied her on the first time she returned to school; thereafter, her parents undertook this responsibility until, after two weeks, she was successfully attending all lessons. At this stage the daily contact via telephone between C and her day unit teacher was withdrawn. Contact with the CAMHS continued over the next school holiday to ensure her attendance progress was maintained.

Refugees and asylum seekers

Children in special circumstances have special needs. Refugee children present with a complex range of emotional and academic needs, and teachers are ideally placed to provide support to a group of children who are often acutely aware of the value of education. Their families may experience a variety of difficulties, from uncertainty about asylum status and the culture shock of living in a new country, to language obstacles or discrimination because of race or immigration status. In the classroom, aggressive, inattentive behaviour or fear of sudden loud noises may be a feature of undiagnosed trauma, part of the syndrome of post-traumatic stress disorder, and this should not be misconstrued as disruptiveness. Many schools are accepting and supportive of refugee children, whereas others may be less understanding and have concerns regarding the effects of speaking English as a second language on school "league" tables. Outreach child mental health services have been successfully offered on primary school sites to refugee children identified by teachers.[13]

Teachers within the health service

Education authorities supply teachers to hospital paediatric wards to teach acutely ill and recovering children. Their role is to maintain each child's academic progress during their hospital stay and follow the school curriculum as far as medical or surgical treatment will allow. Teachers within tiers three and four (see Box 11.1, p. 158) specialist psychiatric settings, such as day and inpatient units, may have an expanded role. Teachers in mental health units have a sophisticated knowledge of child development and educational deficits, as well as the skill to provide therapeutic input. Where local authorities provide education resources it is essential that there is agreement over the priorities of their work. This is usually to maintain children and young people within a mainstream setting. Given the complex nature of teaching within a mental health setting, consideration should perhaps be given to dual training qualifications for this role.

References

1 Rutter M, Maudhan B, Mortimore P, Ouston J. *Fifteen thousand hours.* London: Open Books, 1979.
2 Yates P, Garralda ME, Higginson I. Paddington Complexity Scale and Health of the Nation outcome scales for children and adolescents. *Br J Psychiatry* 1999;**174**: 417–23.
3 Goodman R. The Strengths and Difficulties Questionnaire: a research note. *J Child Psychol Psychiatry* 1997;**38**:581–6.
4 Conners CK. Rating scales for use in drug studies with children. In *Special issue: pharmacotherapy of children. Psychopharmacol Bull* 1973;24–84.
5 Department for Education and Employment. *SEN code of practice on the identification and assessment of pupils with special educational needs.* London: Department for Education and Employment, 2000.
6 Barkley RA. Attention deficit hyperactivity disorder. In: *A clinical workbook.* New York: Guilford Press, 1991:73–7.
7 Overmeyer S, Taylor E. Annotation: principles of treatment of hyperkinetic disorder. Practice approaches for the UK. *J Child Psychol Psychiatry* 1999;**40**: 1147–57.
8 Stevenson J. *Hyperactivity disorders of childhood.* Cambridge: Cambridge University Press, 1996:382–432.
9 McMahon R. Initial impact of the fast track prevention trial for conduct problems II. Classroom effects. *J Consult Clin Psychol* 1999;**67**:648–57.
10 Department for Education and Employment. *Social inclusion: pupil support.* London: Department for Education and Employment, 1999.
11 Olweus D. Bully/victim problems among schoolchildren: basic facts and effects of a school based intervention programme. In: Rubin K, Pepler D, eds. *The development and treatment of childhood aggression.* Hillsdale, NJ: Lawrence Erlbaum, 1991.
12 Blagg N. *School phobia and its treatment.* London: Croom Helm, 1987.
13 O'Shea B, Hodes M, Down G, Bramley J. A school based mental health service for refugee children. *Clin Child Psychol Psychiatry* 2000;5:189–201.

Section IV
Legal aspects

14: Consent and confidentiality

MICHAEL SHAW

Overview

Clinicians try to strike a balance between autonomy and protection when involving young people in decisions about their health care.

Young people are entitled to privacy, information, and a level of decision making geared to their maturity.

Most young people prefer to share treatment decisions with their parents,[1] but some will wish to exclude their parents or oppose their parents' and/or clinician's recommendations.

Every effort should be made to achieve consensus, including providing more time and information or an independent second opinion.

Where agreement is not possible the law usually provides more than one approach to avoid deadlock. The challenge is choosing which legal framework is most appropriate to the circumstances of the particular case.

Introduction

The importance of taking into account the child's views about his or her illness and treatment is increasingly being recognised. This is especially pertinent in adolescence, when the developmentally appropriate experimentation with autonomy and independence from parental protection and authority may spill into clinical decision making.

In practice, clinicians may find themselves having to strike a balance between autonomy and protection when involving young people in decisions about their health care. The way in which this is resolved will centre round themes such as confidentiality, competence, consent or refusal by parents and children to have specific investigations and treatments, and the legal framework for these decisions.

This chapter uses examples of clinical issues to describe these dilemmas and to outline guidelines that may be used to resolve them in practice.

Confidentiality

A number of key points should be noted with respect to confidentiality, and these are listed in Box 14.1.

> ### Box 14.1 Confidentiality: key points
>
> Confidentiality allows patients to trust clinicians with personal information.
> All young people are entitled to confidentiality.
> Protecting young people from risk will sometimes justify breaching confidentiality.
> Parents may have to be informed because only competent young people can consent.
> Advanced warning of the limits of confidentiality or a breach of confidence is part of respecting young people's autonomy.

Case example

A 14 year old girl admitted to hospital with an episode of abdominal pain says that she does not want to go home and hints at abuse by her father. The parents complain about the hospital and demand to see the daughter's notes. The girl is very reluctant to let this happen.

General principles

Trust

It is sometimes necessary for patients to share highly personal details with their clinician. Confidentiality protects the patient from embarrassment and is an important source of patients' trust in clinicians. Patients expect to retain control over personal information and to be asked for permission if that information is used to benefit others (for example, in research or teaching).

Risk

Mental health problems such as anorexia nervosa, substance abuse, or deliberate self harm put young people at risk. Sharing information with a protective third person reduces some risks. The benefit of such protection has to be offset against the cost of breaching trust.

Competence

Young people are entitled to confidentiality whether they are competent or not.[2] However, only competent young people can consent to treatment, and so parents may have to be involved and provided with enough information to make a decision.[3]

Applications

Advanced warning

Young people know what to expect if they are warned about the limits to confidentiality at the start of a consultation. I tell patients

200

that our discussion remains "private" unless I am worried about keeping someone "safe" or require their parent's "permission" to do something. I stress that I would warn them before divulging any information. (See the toolkit developed by the Royal College of General Practitioners and others.[4])

Patients should also be warned that clinicians working in teams may need to share information with their colleagues.

Breaching confidentiality

Advanced warning softens the blow of breaching confidentiality. The young person may come to accept the need to share information, or take comfort in choosing the manner in which information is shared. At the very least they have an opportunity to prepare themselves. Only very rarely will pressure of time or the need for secrecy prevent telling patients before confidentiality is breached.

Response to case example

Returning to the 14 year old girl who is refusing to give her parents access to her medical records, it may be possible to address the concerns of the girl and her parents by further enquiry and discussion. However, the files might be withheld from the parents if the girl was judged competent to make that decision.

Competence

Issues pertaining to competence among young people are summarised in Box 14.2.

Box 14.2 Competence: key points

Competence requires adequate information.
The value of information is increased by an opportunity to ask questions and time to think.
Competence requires young people to:
"understand fully what is proposed"
retain an understanding
appreciate the importance of information and see how it applies to themselves.
weigh information "in the balance".
The level of understanding that is "sufficient" will vary with the complexity and gravity of the decision.
Young people's competence can be:
enhanced by support
impaired by mental or physical states
undermined by coercion.
Judgements about competence can only be made on a case-by-case basis.
In complex cases it is best practice to involve an independent clinician.

Case example

A 15 year old young man with a history of attention deficit/ hyperactivity disorder has been taking methylphenidate for the past eight years; he presents to your general practice asking to stop his medication.

General principles

Introduction

Whether or not a young person is competent to make a particular treatment decision varies with the availability of information and time, their level of understanding, the complexity and gravity of the decision, their ability to think about the issues, and the presence of factors that enhance or impair these capacities.

Information and time

Competence is only possible in the presence of adequate information. The guidelines from the General Medical Council[5] and British Medical Association (BMA)[6] both stress the importance of providing adequate information. The value of information will be increased by an opportunity to ask questions and (in the absence of an overriding need to act) time to "sleep on" a decision.

Understanding

Ruling in the Gillick case (see below), Lord Scarman linked competence to "sufficient understanding and intelligence" to allow a young person "to understand fully what is proposed". Understanding "fully" includes understanding the nature of the condition/illness, the investigation and treatment procedures, the benefits and risks of treatments, the treatment options, and the outlook with or without treatment.

Complexity and gravity of the decision

The level of understanding that is "sufficient" will vary with the complexity and gravity of the decision. Of particular importance are the relative benefits, risks, and burdens of treatment options. Greater understanding is expected if the burdens are heavy, the risks high, or the benefits uncertain. Similarly, a higher level of understanding is required if young people refuse treatment.[7]

Building on understanding

Justice Thorpe's decision in Re C (adult: refusal of medical treatment)[8] broadens the Gillick concept of competence. C was a patient at Broadmoor Hospital suffering from schizophrenia who refused amputation of his gangrenous foot. Ruling that C should decide for himself, the court defined competence as "first comprehending and retaining information, secondly, believing it and thirdly, weighing it in the balance to arrive at a choice". In this context "believing" means the young person appreciates the importance of information and sees how it applies to them. A young person may weigh the information differently from their parents or doctor, and unwise choices might be permitted.

Finally when evaluating young people's competence it is important not to set a higher standard than would be expected for adults.

Enhancing competence

Young people's competence will be enhanced if they feel loved and supported. Most people prefer to discuss important decisions with a family member or friend. Equally, discussion with health professionals will be more productive when the relationship is founded on trust and respect.

Threats to competence

Competence can be temporarily impaired by certain mental or physical states. Mental illness may impair a young person's judgement sufficiently that they are rendered incompetent, but it is important not to assume that all (or even most) mentally ill people are incompetent. Finally, competence can be undermined by coercion from peers, family, or even health professionals.

Applications

Judgements about competence can only be made case by case, taking account of the individual, the type of decision and the particular circumstances. The BMA guidance on consent in young people[6] (pages 101–103 in that document) provides an excellent list of practical ways to enhance competence. In complex cases it is best practice for an independent clinician to advise on competence and vital to document any decision about competence.

Responding to the case example

Returning to the 15 year old boy who wants to stop his medication, discussing the options and assessing his competence will help to decide how to proceed. The first step is to ensure that he is fully informed about his condition and its treatment. Next, we need to assess his ability to understand, retain, apply, and weigh the information in the balance. Finally, it is necessary to assess factors that may be influencing his level of competence.

Consent

Key points regarding consent are summarised in Box 14.3. Furthermore, ruling in the Gillick case,[9] Lord Fraser set out five preconditions that would justify treating an individual under 16 years old without his or her parents' consent (see below).

Box 14.3 Consent: key points

Outside of emergencies or the Mental Health Act 1983, consent is a prerequisite to treatment.

Consent is the voluntary and continuing permission to receive a particular treatment, based on an adequate knowledge.

A person with parental responsibility can give consent on behalf of the young person.

If a 16 or 17 year old consents, it is unnecessary to seek consent from a person with parental responsibility.

A competent person under 16 has an independent right to consent to treatment; however, it is good practice to also seek consent from a person with parental responsibility.

Case example

A 14 year old boy presents to your general practice requesting anti-depressants. He has a four-month history of depressive symptoms with increasing suicidal thoughts. He insists that his parents are not informed.

General principles

The law

Other than for emergencies or in the circumstances described in part IV of the Mental Health Act 1983, consent is a necessary prerequisite to the treatment of any young person. The Department of Health's code of practice with regard to the Act[10] gives the following definition of consent (15.13): "'Consent' is the voluntary and continuing permission of the patient to receive a particular treatment, based on an adequate knowledge of the purpose, nature, likely effects and risks of that treatment including the likelihood of its success and any alternatives to it. Permission given under any unfair undue pressure is not 'consent'."

The General Medical Council guidance on consent[5] places particular emphasis on providing patients with adequate information and freedom from pressure.

A person with parental responsibility (including a local authority with a care order) can give consent on behalf of the young person (before their 18th birthday). However, this power is subject to a number of qualifications.

Those aged 16 or 17. The Family Law Reform Act 1969 lowered the age of majority to 18 years, and gave 16 and 17 year olds the same right of consent as adults (s8 [1]). This means that if a 16 or 17 year old person consents, then it is unnecessary to seek consent from a person with parental responsibility. (However, see the section on refusal, below.)

Those under 16. As described above, the competence of a young person under the age of 16 years is considered in light of the Gillick decision. This ruling gives under 16 year olds with sufficient understanding ("Gillick competent") an independent right to consent to treatment. However, even with a Gillick competent young person (under the age of 16 years), it is good practice also to seek consent from a person with parental responsibility. In his ruling in the Gillick case, Lord Fraser set out five preconditions that would justify a doctor prescribing contraceptives to a young woman under the age of 16 years without her parents' consent:

- that the girl (although under the age of 16 years) will understand the doctor's advice
- that the doctor cannot persuade her to inform her parents or to allow him to inform the parents that she is seeking contraceptive advice
- that she is very likely to begin or to continue having sexual intercourse with or without contraceptive treatment
- that unless she receives contraceptive advice or treatment, her physical and mental health or both are likely to suffer
- that her best interests require the doctor to give her contraceptive advice or treatment, or both, without parental consent.

Although there is no lower age limit, Bailey and Harbour[11] suggested that it would rarely be appropriate for a young person under the age of 13 years to consent to treatment without their parent's involvement.

Applications

There are many reasons for informing children and gaining their cooperation over and above obtaining valid consent. Alderson[1] cites the following reasons: out of respect for the child; to answer questions and help the child to know what to expect; to reduce anxiety; to help the child make sense of their experience; to warn about risks; to prevent misunderstanding or resentment; to promote confidence and courage; and to increase compliance.

Responding to the case example

Returning to the depressed 14 year old boy and the question of whether he can receive antidepressants without his parent's consent, this young man should be treated without his parent's consent if he is competent, cannot be persuaded to involve his parents, and would be at risk if treatment were withheld. There may be someone else he can confide in who could be involved in his treatment, and he may feel more comfortable involving his parents once his mood improves.

Refusal

Key points in refusal are summarised in Box 14.4.

Box 14.4 Refusal: key points

Unlike the competent adult, the competent child's wishes may be overruled in pursuit of his or her welfare.

The consent of a person with parental responsibility will override the refusal of the young person (whether they are competent or not).

Every effort should be made to reach a consensus, including provision of more information and time, or the involvement of an independent second opinion.

It is sometimes necessary to override the objections of a young person who is likely to suffer significant harm without treatment.

The Mental Health Act 1983 goes further than common law to protect the rights of young people treated against their wishes and may be used to treat people of any age.

In Scotland, competent minors have an independent right to consent to or refuse treatment.

Occasionally, the court needs to intervene in situations in which parents withhold treatment.

Where children have been abused or neglected by their parents, it is inappropriate to use parental authority to override the child's objections.

Case example

At a routine paediatric outpatient appointment, a 12 year old girl with insulin dependent diabetes mellitus presents unwell with a five-month history of restricted calorie intake, excessive exercising, and 10 kg weight loss; despite being painfully thin, she wants to lose more weight. She refuses to come into hospital and see a psychiatrist.

General principles

The law

A competent adult has a right to refuse treatment "for reasons which are rational or irrational, or for no reason".[12] The Children Act explicitly gives those who are competent and under 16 years old the right to refuse assessment and treatment in the very limited circumstances of care proceedings (which can be overridden by the court). The Act and accompanying guidance and regulations place considerable emphasis on taking account of the child's views. However, the central premise of the Children Act is that "the child's welfare shall be the court's paramount consideration" (s1 [1]). Unlike the competent adult, the competent child's views may be overruled in pursuit of his or her welfare.

Furthermore two rulings by the Court of Appeal (Re R[13] and Re W[14]) significantly curtail a young person's ability to refuse treatment. They concern R, a 15 year old young woman refusing antipsychotic medication, and W, a 16 year old young woman with anorexia nervosa refusing transfer to another treatment centre. In both cases the Court of Appeal ruled that treatment could lawfully proceed with the consent of either a competent young person or a person with parental responsibility, and that the consent of a person with parental responsibility would override the refusal of the young person.

There are other situations in which the competent young person can be overruled. When they are in care, the local authority has parental responsibility and can give consent (parents retain responsibility, and it is good practice to consult them). Young people who are wards of court can only receive treatment with the leave of the court, and the court can use its inherent jurisdiction to overrule a competent child.

Where someone with parental responsibility gives consent but a competent young person refuses, there are circumstances in which it is still advisable to obtain the authority of the court (p. 38 of the BMA document).[6] The BMA recommends that, outside of emergencies, the court's approval should be sought for any treatment that involves the restraint or detention of a competent young person (ibid p. 114). In cases that involve sterilisation or abortion, the court's guidance should always be sought. If neither the young person nor any other person can give valid consent, then the authority of the court should be sought. (See ibid p. 50 for a discussion of the circumstances in which it is appropriate to seek legal advice.) It would usually be inappropriate for a parent who has abused his or her child to give consent on that child's behalf. Where the young person is not already in the care of the local authority, the court's authority should be sought.

Parents have a duty under the Children and Young Persons Act 1933 5 (I) to obtain essential medical assistance for a child under the age of 16. Occasionally, the court needs to intervene in situations in which parents withhold treatment. Where the parent's refusal is part of a wider process of neglect or abuse, a care order may be appropriate. This gives the local authority parental responsibility, and treatment can proceed with their consent. If the parent's care of the child is generally satisfactory and their objection to treatment is on the basis of religious or other strongly held beliefs, it is possible to ask the High Court to use its inherent jurisdiction to overrule the parents, or apply for a specific issue order.

The Mental Health Act 1983 may be used to treat people of any age. With its requirement for a second opinion, time limited application, and opportunity for independent review, the Mental Health Act goes further than common law to protect the rights of young people treated against their wishes. However, there is still a stigma attached to being detained under the Mental Health Act. My view is that, in situations where the Mental Health Act would normally apply, it should be preferred. (For a full comparison of the two legal frameworks, see White et al.,[15] and Bailey and Harbour 1999.[11])

In Scotland competent minors have an independent right to consent to or refuse treatment (the Age of Legal Capacity [Scotland] Act 1991).

Applications

Provided that delay does not lead to unacceptable risks, every effort should be made to reach consensus.[7] The BMA[6] suggests that another health professional be asked to act as an independent arbiter and attempt to negotiate an agreement.

I believe that no young person (competent or otherwise) should be treated against their will unless they are more likely than not to suffer significant harm without treatment. Even when overruling a young person's refusal, it will often be possible to give limited choices.

See the guidelines for good practice on consent listed in Box 14.5,[16] which attempts to build upon the best features of the law and guidance in this area.

Box 14.5 Guidelines for good practice on consent (modified from Shaw[16] with permission)

Parents and young people (whether or not they are competent) must be informed and involved as much as possible in treatment decisions.

Treatment can proceed with the consent of a person with parental responsibility and the incompetent young person's agreement, or the competent young person's consent.

If either the parent or young person refuses, then treatment should be delayed for more discussion, modification of the treatment plan, or the help of an independent arbiter.

(Continued)

Treatment may proceed with the consent of one person with parental responsibility (Children Act, s2 [7]), even if there is opposition from another. The onus is on that person to obtain a prohibited steps order under section 8.

If there is no person with parental responsibility who is willing to consent to necessary action or treatment programme for a child who is not competent, then consideration must be given to obtaining a specific issue order or asking the local authority to seek a care order.

Overruling the refusal of any young person (competent or not) should only be considered if:

discussion and modification of the treatment have been exhausted

(and) the parents are in favour or the authority of the court is obtained

(and) the young person is more likely than not to suffer significant harm without treatment.

Before treating a young person against his or her will:

consider whether treatment under the Mental Health Act is indicated

alternatively, the decision should be confirmed by a second opinion

(and) a time limit set for reviewing the decision

(and) the reasons for the decision should be recorded in the notes.

If it is considered necessary to overrule the refusal of consent by a competent child, then legal advice should be taken on whether to rely on the consent of a person with parental responsibility, if available, or whether to seek the authority of the court.

Parents or the young person can withdraw consent at any time.

Staff need to be aware of the service's policy on consent.

Staff will need training and ongoing support to achieve an appropriate balance between autonomy and protection.

Response to the case example

Returning to the 12 year old girl with diabetes and weight loss, every effort should be made to help this young woman understand the danger she is in and take steps to make herself safe. She probably has an eating disorder and/or depression, and if necessary she could be treated against her will under the Mental Health Act. If her refusal were felt to be because she was too young to understand the issues, then it might be more appropriate to treat her under common law. Were she to suddenly lapse into hypoglycaemic coma, emergency treatment would not require consent, but once out of danger consent would be needed for any further investigation or treatment.

References

1   Alderson P. *Children's consent to surgery*. Buckingham: Open University Press, 1993.
2   Royal College of Psychiatrists. *Good psychiatric practice: confidentiality. Council report CR85*. London: The Royal College of Psychiatrists, 2000.
3   Department of Health. *Seeking consent: working with children*. London: Department of Health, 2001.

4 Royal College of General Practitioners, Brook, General Practitioners Committee, British Medical Association, Royal College of Nursing, and Medical Defence Union. *Confidentiality and young people. Improving teenagers' uptake of sexual and other health advice.* London: The Royal College of General Practitioners, 2000.

5 General Medical Council. *Seeking patients' consent: the ethical considerations.* London: General Medical Council, 1999.

6 British Medical Association. *Consent, rights and choices in health care for children and young people.* London: BMA, 2001.

7 Pearce J. Consent to treatment during childhood: the assessment of competence and avoidance of conflict. *Br J Psychiatry* 1994;**165**:713–6.

8 Re C (adult: refusal of treatment) [1994] 1 FLR 31.

9 Gillick v West Norfolk and Wisbech Area Health Authority [1986] AC 112.

10 Department of Health and Welsh Office. *Code of practice: Mental Health Act 1983.* London: HMSO, 1999.

11 Bailey P, Harbour A. The law and a child's consent to treatment (England and Wales). *Child Psychol Psychiatry Rev* 1999;**4**:30–4.

12 Sidaway v Board of Governors of the Bethlem Royal Hospital and the Maudsley Hospital [1985] AC 871.

13 Re R (a minor) (wardship: medical treatment) [1992] Fam 11, [1991] 4 All ER 177, CA.

14 Re W (a minor) (wardship: medical treatment) [1993] Fam 64, [1992] 4 All ER 627, CA.

15 White R, Williams R, Harbour A, Bingley W. *Safeguards for young minds: young people and protective legislation.* London: Gaskell, 1996.

16 Shaw M. Childhood, mental health and the law. In: Green J, Jacobs B, eds. *In-patient child psychiatry: modern practice, research and the future.* London: Routledge, 1998.

15: Parenting breakdown and the courts

CLAIRE STURGE

Overview

Parenting is central to the welfare of children.

Parenting failure and its consequences present to mental health professionals in a variety of ways.

Parenting breakdown can cause significant harm to a child or put the child at risk of such harm.

Parenting failures can be acts of commission such as abuse (physical, sexual or emotional).

Child and adolescent mental health services are often needed to assess the parenting of a child and how it meets the needs of a particular child.

These professionals may be instructed as experts in advising the courts on parenting issues.

Introduction

Parenting impacts on child psychiatric practice in important ways. Assessment and management in child and adolescent psychiatry rely almost universally on collaboration between clinicians, parents, and children. Moreover, for a number of children with problems of psychiatric adjustment, poor parenting or family breakdown may be central in the aetiology of the child's disorder, or may impede parental ability to reduce adverse consequences for the child. Society invests in the legal system a responsibility for safeguarding the best interests of children. Child psychiatrists and legal professionals are sometimes required to work together toward ensuring that a child's mental health needs are attended to safely and appropriately. This chapter discusses issues over which the courts are likely to seek the expertise of the child and adolescent psychiatrist.

Private and public law

Courts are principally involved with children either when parents separate and bring matters such as residence or contact before the

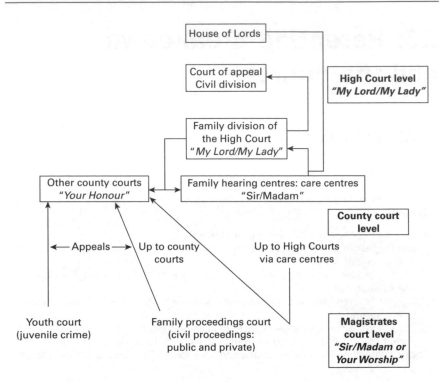

Figure 15.1 Court structures

court, or where the local authority intervenes by seeking an order through the courts because it believes the child is suffering or is likely to suffer from harm. The former types of cases are referred to as private law and the latter as public law cases. Both types of proceedings come under the remit of the Children Act 1989. This chapter will deal mainly with the public law issues but starts by briefly looking at private law. For reference, court structures are briefly summarised in Figure 15.1.

Private law

The issues

In the majority of cases in which parents separate, arrangements about future care and sharing of care for children are decided by mutual agreement.

A parent can apply to court to seek residence of the child or specific contact arrangements. This applies whether the parents were married or not. Usually, if the father does not have parental responsibility because the child was born outside wedlock, he will seek to gain this early in legal proceedings. By definition, in any case reaching court the parents have failed to resolve matters and are in dispute. In such cases there are often allegations and counter allegations involving complaints that range from unreliability over contact to allegations of domestic violence, abuse, or neglect of children, or concerns about the mental health of a parent or worries about problems arising out of intoxication with alcohol or drugs.

Most private law cases are managed by magistrates and county courts, although the most complex reach the High Court. An officer from the Children and Families Court Advisory and Support Service (CAFCASS) will usually explore the child's circumstances for the court and experts such as child psychiatrists or clinical psychologists are only instructed when there are complex issues.

CAFCASS is a new service that resulted from the amalgamation of a range of officers working on behalf of children and families in the court system. Guardians ad litem, court welfare officers, the Child Care arm of the Official Solicitors Department, and probation officers involved in family work are now all subsumed under this title. There have been various difficulties in setting up the new service but these are expected to be resolved in time.

The court makes decisions based on the best interests of the child and can make residence and contact orders in respect of the child and a particular parent. It can also make specific issues orders, for example regarding medical treatment or the school a child should attend.

Approximately 100,000 applications in respect of residence and contact are made each year in England and Wales, and these (being mostly legally aided) cost the Exchequer an enormous amount of money.

Contribution of child and adolescent psychiatrists/mental health services

The area of private law is important for child mental health practice because there is considerable evidence of the ill effects of parental separation on children and their emotional wellbeing, particularly where this is acrimonious. Numerically, parental separation can be seen as the single most important variable in children's lives, possibly determining the short and long term emotional outcome for hundreds of thousands of children.[1-3]

Issues on which a court might seek the expertise of a child mental health specialist include the following:

- assessment of the child's mental state and his or her relationship with each parent
- assessment of allegations of abuse

Table 15.1 Courts: civil proceedings concerning children and adolescents in magistrates' and county courts, and high courts

Issues	Parties	Range of orders or directions
Parenting breakdown, including abuse and being beyond parental control	Social services and others, for example grandparents	Resident, contact, supervision and care orders, specific directions
School non-attendance	Education authority, parents	Education supervision order
Marital breakdown	Between parents	Residence orders, contact orders, specific issues/prohibitive steps orders
Welfare and consent issues, such as child abduction and treatment refusal	Any	Inherent jurisdiction of the High Court/wardship, Children Act orders (High Court)
Challenges about statutory services, for example services to a "child in need"	Any: particularly parents versus education, social services, or health authorities	Judicial review: decisions are binding on parties

- assessment of the impact of the parental disputes, including past disputes involving alleged or proven domestic violence on the child
- determination of the relevance of any of these factors to questions of where the child should live or what type of contact he should have with the non-resident parent.

An important issue to consider in contact disputes is what purpose the contact can serve for the child. The type (indirect or direct, supervised or unsupervised), frequency, and duration of the contact will be determined by its purpose, taking into account the developmental stage and the particular circumstances of the individual child.

It is unusual for social services to be involved in such cases, but they may be asked to make an assessment (section 7 or 37 of the Children Act 1989) or to report if they are or have been involved with the family. The court can, with the local authority's agreement, make a section 7 order, requiring social services to assist the family for a period of up to one year.

The circumstances in which a range of court orders or directions can be given, as well as the parties involved, are summarised in Table 15.1.

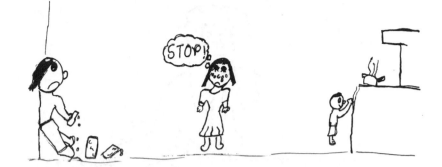

"Mum's been drinking." Children may become deeply despondent about responsibilities imposed on them by a major breakdown in parenting

Public law

The issues

A local authority usually brings cases in which a care or supervision order, an adoption order, or a child assessment order may be sought. Wardship or the inherent jurisdiction of the High Court can also be sought by any party, including providers of health services, but this is now very rare.

Parents can oppose applications for care or supervision orders. They can seek to have them discharged or can apply to obtain or vary contact arrangements.

In cases of parenting breakdown, in which a case is brought to court because of concerns that the parenting is failing to meet the child's needs or there is considered to be an ongoing risk for abuse or neglect, then a comprehensive assessment is sought by the courts. This usually involves a multiagency approach involving social services, health, and, occasionally, education.

A child who is beyond parental control represents additional grounds for making a care or supervision order. When the Adoption and Children Act 2002 is enacted, exposure to domestic violence, direct or indirect, will also be considered to constitute significant harm.

Contribution of child and adolescent psychiatrists/mental health services

Experts are now more frequently brought in than not. Such assessments can be seen as specialist assessments, as defined by the new "Framework for the Assessment of Children in Need and their Families".[4] Under the new Framework, such assessments can be built on the foundation of the core assessment coordinated by the local authority. Any parenting assessment needs careful planning and

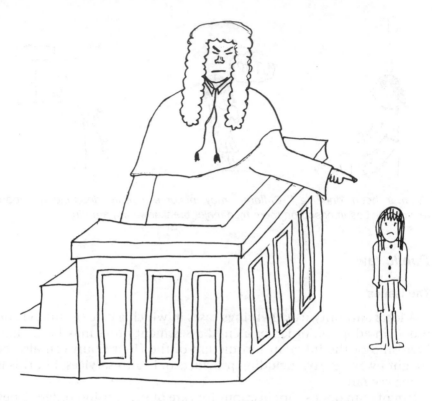

In the best interests of the child, the court attempts to choose the least detrimental option

usually requires interagency input, involving health and education services, as well as social services. The aim is to conduct the assessment in partnership with parents but it is often difficult for a parent to contribute to assessment planning in an objective manner. Ideally, assessments for courts should be planned jointly with all agencies involved, with a high level of collaboration, and, where appropriate, joint or complementary assessments.

The importance of parenting

Parenting is the "how" of how parents bring up their children. It is a complex and difficult task. Awareness is increasing of the importance of different patterns of parenting. Associations between certain parenting patterns and particular problems for the child are now recognised. The importance of parental warmth and approval for children's healthy emotional development has been identified for nearly half a century.[5] More recently, the role of different styles of

Table 15.2 Parenting assessment: the child's basic needs	
Child's need	Details
Security/safety	Safety: food, warmth, clothing, etc., and home, car, road, personal safety
	Security: sense of safety necessary for security; stability and consistency of care givers, care itself, discipline, and boundaries. Mutual trust. Sense of being listened to and good channels of communication. Perception of parents as strong, able to cope, being in control, responsive
Belongingness	Continuity of care givers. Clear identity, for example names, roots, culture. Sense of permanence. Personal or individual space and possessions
Self actualisation/ identity development	Child treated as special and unique. Child seen as separate from parent by the parent(s) (distinction of needs). Perceptiveness of child's individuality and particular needs. Lack of intrusiveness
Praise/esteem	Meeting of child's need for esteem and praise. Expression of warmth and positive feelings, absence of hostility. Appropriate positive reinforcement. Valuing the child's "differentness"
New experience/ knowledge	Encouragement of learning, extending new experiences and independence. Giving child a sense of responsibility for his or her actions and for their impact on others

parenting has been studied, and supervision and warmth – or lack thereof – in parent–child relationships have been linked to antisocial behaviours. Although very early parent–child relationships, including attachment, are known to be important in a child's overall development, knowledge is not detailed enough for specific predictions to be made.

All children have a range of physical, emotional, social, and educational needs (for summary, see Table 15.2). Abuse and neglect can be seen as a significant failure to meet a child's needs in one of these areas. If the failure is in relation to the child's psychological needs, then this can be termed psychological abuse or emotional neglect or abuse. The difficulty is, of course, in determining the dividing line between the weaknesses to be found in most parenting and the point at which this amounts to significant abuse or neglect.

Parenting breakdown

Parental separation and divorce can be seen as a form of parenting breakdown, but this chapter focuses more on the parenting breakdown identified specifically through concerns about the child.

Table 15.3 Parenting breakdown

Problem/concern	Main focus for assessment in addition to parenting
Physical abuse	Paediatric assessment: risk to health and life, emotional damage
Sexual abuse	Non-abusing parent's ability to support and protect the child. Child's emotional state and needs, treatment needs
Failure to thrive; physical deprivation	Paediatric assessment
Emotional abuse, emotional deprivation	Child's emotional state and needs, treatment needs
Factitious disorder	Paediatric assessment: risk to health and life. Psychiatric assessment of parent
Parental mental disorder: mental illness, personality disorder, substance abuse, mental handicap	Psychiatric/psychology assessment, with particular reference to ability to make responsible decisions and prognosis
Beyond control: usually adolescents	Assessment of youngster's needs

In this sense, parenting breakdown can be seen as any of the following (Table 15.3):

- a parent seeks to have their child removed, often because the child, usually an adolescent, is beyond their control or when the parent cannot cope for other reasons, including a lack of commitment to the child
- the child is abandoned
- child abuse or neglect is proved or suspected; this can take the form of physical or emotional neglect or physical, sexual, or emotional abuse. Usually, more than one form is seen in combination, and all forms of abuse involve elements of emotional abuse.

The assessment of parenting

Where significant concerns are identified in relation to parenting, the nature of the problems must be assessed. The aim of such an assessment will be to identify what the problems are and what types of intervention would ameliorate them. The conclusion may be that

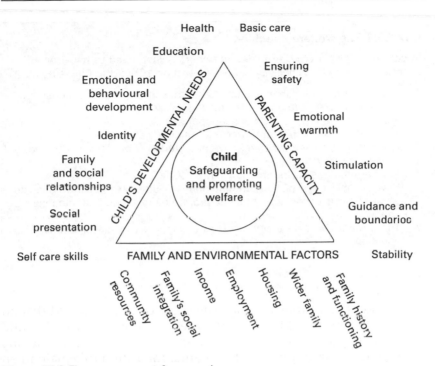

Figure 15.2 The assessment framework

the problems are too serious or any period of remediation would be outside of time scales appropriate to the child, and that the child should be provided with alternative care.

The "Framework for the Assessment of Children in Need and their Families"[4] is the newly introduced guideline for assessing a child's situation comprehensively and includes examination of parenting (Figure 15.2). The comprehensive assessment in this scheme may then lead on to specialist assessment. This is nearly always the case where care proceedings are planned or already in progress.

In court proceedings the requirements of an assessment take on a more specific form related to the law. The court will want to know whether the child has suffered harm or is likely to suffer harm; what evidence there is for this; and whether it is attributable to the care given by the parent (when compared with what one might reasonably expect of a parent). The court will then decide whether this amounts to significant harm (the "threshold criteria") and make decisions for the child based on principles of the paramount importance of the child and of his or her welfare (hence the "welfare checklist" – see Box 15.1).

Box 15.1 The welfare checklist

In considering what order to make, the court is instructed to have regard in particular to a welfare checklist set out in section 1(3) of the Children Act.

1. The ascertainable wishes and feelings of the child concerned (considered in the light of his age and understanding).
2. His physical, emotional and educational needs.
3. The likely effect on him of any change of circumstances.
4. His age, sex background, and any characteristics of his which the court considers relevant.
5. Any harm he has suffered or is likely to suffer.
6. How capable each of his parents, and any other person in relation to whom the court considered the question to be relevant, is of meeting his needs.
7. The powers available to the court under this Act in the proceedings in question.

In considering making an order, the court must be satisfied that an order is better for the child than no order. All those involved in child care are acutely aware of the risks encountered by children in the care system, and that it may be less detrimental for a child to remain in an unsatisfactory home situation than to be removed.

Care and supervision orders can be made by a court where evidence of significant harm (or its likelihood) attributable to the care received from the parents is proved and an order is in the child's interests. On occasion, hearings are split, with the first hearing dealing with the question of whether the threshold of significant harm is met and the second dealing with plans for the children consequent to the finding in the first and further assessment of options for planning. This can be useful when, initially, all of the parents' energies are invested in disproving any allegations, and when they cannot move on to considering interventions and the future while they are so narrowly preoccupied.

Areas for consideration in a specialist assessment

The following comprise the main categories under which detailed assessment needs to be undertaken[6]:

- the parent's relationship to the role of parenting; this includes attitudes, style, and skills
- the parent's relationship with the child
- family influences, including the parent's own experience of being parented and relationships with those parents; the current parenting relationship

- interaction with the outside world, including general ability to cope and support networks
- potential for change.

Which of the above is emphasised in the assessment will depend on the central issues identified. These will vary. For example, where the parent has a mental illness, the same outline is followed but a specific focus, within the parent's relationship to the child domain, may be whether the child is part of the parent's delusional system or the target of hostility. With a learning disabled parent, the assessment again follows the same lines but the extent to which the child's needs are met is more important than assumptions based on parental IQ.

The potential for change is often the most challenging part of an assessment. Some indication can be gleaned from past experiences with the family: levels of cooperation; response and attitude to previous interventions; periods when family functioning was better; and acknowledgement and acceptance of responsibility for problems. The most satisfactory way to assess this is to implement an intervention and measure change. The parent–child game (a particularly detailed technique to assess parent–child interactions) is designed to do this but, time allowing, there are a range of approaches to address this question.

A court may request an assessment from a specialist in order to obtain an expert opinion. Unlike a professional witness who reports within the confines of their clinical involvement with a case, the duty of an expert witness is to the court and lies in providing an opinion on matters that the court has instructed him or her to address.

The topic of parenting and its assessment cannot be fully covered in a chapter. A case example may help to illustrate basic principles.

Case example

Oscar was eight and his brother Liam was three. Oscar was taken into care on an emergency protection order when he was found wandering the streets. Liam was removed later the same day when he was found being cared for by friends who reported that he had been left with them following a fight between the parents the previous day.

Preliminary enquiries indicated that the parental couple were well known to the police in relation to domestic violence. Oscar had been in extreme difficulties in school with his aggressive behaviour and had been suspended several times. No concerns were identified in relation to Liam.

The family had been known to a social services department in another area, and information from that department indicated that the mother had had a very disrupted childhood. On the positive side, the parents had been successful educationally and in their work.

An interagency parenting assessment planning meeting identified the following as particular areas for detailed assessment:

- the parental relationship and violence
- the prognosis in relation to the domestic violence and what interventions might be effective (i.e. ability to change)
- an assessment of the children, with particular reference to Oscar's behaviour problems and their likely cause
- Oscar's perceptions and views
- the parent–child relationships, and the nature of any attachment and other aspects of the relationships
- support networks, including assessment of what the extended family might be able to offer.

Clinical psychologists with experience in domestic violence were commissioned to assess the first two points; Child and Adolescent Mental Health Services (CAMHS) and family centre workers undertook the assessment of third, fourth, and fifth items. The field social worker coordinated the assessments and looked at the last item. The areas to be assessed in this case, along with the agencies involved, are summarised in Table 15.4.

The outcome of the assessment was that some potential for change was identified and interim arrangements were recommended for the children while interventions with the parents were tested out.

Table 15.4 Requirements for the assessment

Areas to be assessed	How/by whom
Children's health, and physical and emotional development. Are any problems attributable to the parenting received?	Child health specialist, child psychiatrist or psychologist
Parenting capacity – jointly and separately, intrafamilial relationships/attachments	Specialist family assessment workers/child psychiatrist or psychologist
Each parent's background: early life and relationships; adult relationships; mental health issues. Nature and likely prognosis of the domestic violence	General or forensic adult psychiatrist or psychologist
The parent's ability to engage with professionals/potential for change	Social services/all professionals
General family circumstances and support networks/alternative carers	Social services
Children's educational needs, particularly Oscar's	Education

Parent–child attachments were strong but there were problems within these and in how the parents dealt with Oscar's difficulties. Both parents had dysfunctional experiences of parenting in their own childhoods, and these influenced their behaviour toward each other, their behaviour as a parenting couple, and their parenting.

Oscar showed some innate vulnerability to impulsive behaviour, but the degree of aggression associated with this was seen to result from the exposure to domestic violence. Parenting work would be done at a later stage (before any rehabilitation) if the parents showed progress in their own therapeutic work. Oscar's difficulties would be monitored and further assessed in the light of a future care placement.

By the time of the final hearing (which had been postponed) a year later, the parents had engaged individually and as a couple in therapy, there had been no further incidents of reported violence, and the quality of contact and commitment to the boys was good. Oscar continued to have difficulties in school and the children were generally unsettled. A rehabilitation programme was agreed, which resulted in the boys' returning home on a supervision order after a period of parent training and family work.

The contribution of Child and Adolescent Mental Health Services to the assessment of parenting

Child and adolescent psychiatrists, and to a lesser extent child psychologists and other child and adolescent mental health specialists, may be heavily involved in court work in relation to parenting. As already stated, in virtually all care proceedings a child mental health expert opinion is sought. The controversial issue is the extent to which this should take place within National Health Service practice. With a dearth of experts, this is a very live issue.

There are also issues of public expense (appointing experts at great cost when the local services, within a multiagency framework, might provide this service for less) and the issue of ownership by local services of treatment and other recommendations made by an unconnected expert knowing little of the local scene. These issues are for government departments, commissioning agencies, and individual CAMHS to resolve.

What can be identified are areas where child and adolescent mental health professionals have particular contributions to make. How unique these are in any locality will depend to an extent on the level of training and expertise in allied services, for example social services and family centres.

Child and adolescent mental health specialists can contribute the following:

- consultation to social services, CAFCASS, and the legal profession about issues that need to be addressed and the structure of assessments
- assessment of the child leading to an opinion on the nature of their problems and the likely cause and meaning of these (i.e. issues concerning significant harm). (In the case of physical injury, failure to thrive, or physical neglect, such opinions will lie within the remit of paediatricians)
- assessment of the quality of parent–child relationships, including attachment in younger children
- the nature of the relationships a parent had with his or her own parents as remembered by them and the relevance of this to their parenting of their children
- in collaboration with others, an assessment of the parent's ability to change (for example, a reassessment following a parenting intervention)
- application of knowledge about the impact of adult mental health problems on children and taking this into account within the assessment
- application of knowledge of specific situations (e.g. a severe disorder in the child such as autism) and the relevance of this to observations made
- offering any research based evidence that may be relevant
- comments and advice to parties about the implications of available assessments.

Conclusion

Parenting is a major environmental variable in our society that affects the healthy development of children. Serious deficits result in harm to children, and this will lead to a requirement for legal involvement. In many cases the situation can be ameliorated with appropriate support and interventions; in some cases, the child will be better off in alternative care.

Because of their background, training and experience, child and adolescent mental health specialists have an important contribution to make in the assessment of parenting problems. Also, they can advise on or offer interventions to improve the child's situation, and are often asked to advise the courts in the most serious situations.

References

1 Wallerstein JS, Corbin SB, Lewis JM. Children of divorce: a ten year study. In: Hetherington EM, Arasteh JD, eds. *Impact of divorce, single parenting and stepparenting on children*. Hillsdale, NJ: Erlbaum, 1988.

2   Amato PR, Keith B. Parental divorce and the well-being of children: a meta-analysis. *Psychol Bull* 1991;**110**:26–46.
3   Rodgers B, Pryor J. *Divorce and separation: the outcomes for children.* York, UK: Joseph Rowntree Foundation, 1998.
4   Department of Health, Department of Education and Employment Home Office. *Framework for the Assessment of Children in Need and their Families.* London: The Stationery Office, 2000.
5   Brown GW, Rutter M. The measurement of family activities and relationships: a methodological study. *Hum Relations* 1966;**19**:241–63.
6   Reder P, Lucey C. Significant issues in the assessment of parenting. In: Reder P, Lucey C, eds. *Assessment of parenting: psychiatric and psychological contributions.* London: Routledge, 1995.

Further reading

Advisory Board of Family Law. *A report to the Lord Chancellor on the question of parental contact in cases where there is domestic violence.* London: The Advisory Board of Family Law, The Children Act Sub-Committee chaired by Justice Nicholas Wall, 1999.
Black D, Harris-Hendricks J, Wolkind S. *Child psychiatry and the law.* London: Gaskell, Royal College of Psychiatrists, 1998.
Sturge C. Contact and domestic violence: the experts' court report. *Family Law* 2000;**30**:615–29. (In consultation with Dr D. Glaser.)
Sturge C. A multi-agency approach to the assessment of parenting. *Child Psychol Psychiatry Rev* 2001;**6**:16–20.
Wall J, Hamilton I. *A handbook for expert witnesses in Children Act cases.* Bristol: Family Law (Jordan Publishing Ltd), 2000.

Index

Page numbers printed in *italics* refer to tables and boxed material. Page numbers printed in **bold** refer to figures. Please note that the following abbreviations have been used as subentries: ADHD, attention deficit hyperactivity disorder; CAMHS, Child and Adolescent Mental Health Services; IPT-A, interpersonal psychotherapy for adolescent depression

residence orders 212–13
reward systems 48
  parenting programmes 36
risk, confidentiality issues 200
risperidone, tics and Tourette
    syndrome treatment 133
role disputes, adolescent
    depression 60
role play, IPT-A 57
role transitions, adolescent
    depression 60–1
Routh Activity Scale 162

scapegoating, psychodynamic group
    therapy 107
schizophrenia
  drug treatment 127–30
    see also neuroleptic drugs
  family therapy 119–20
"School Action" 189
"School Action Plus" 189–90
school age children, psychiatric
    disorders and 10–11, *11*
school nurses 162–3
school refusal 52, 193–4
  drug treatment 134–5
schools
  anti bullying package 164
  CAMHS and 186–95
    assessments *188*, 188–9
    contacts 187, *187*
    special educational needs
        189–92, **190**
    see also learning disabilities
  disruptive behaviour 192–3
  influence on pupil behaviour
      186–7
  IPT-A, role in 61–2
  nurses' role 162–3
  refugees and asylum seekers 194
  role in psychiatric aetiology 6
  see also education; school refusal
"scripts," family therapy 116
seasonal affective disorder (SAD),
    treatment 132
self-esteem
  protective role 7
  psychodynamic group
      therapy 104

self harm
  confidentiality issues 200
  drug treatment 142
  group therapy intervention 92
  incidence 175
self help parenting programmes 41
self-monitoring, core cognitive
    techniques 48, 49
"self-talk"
  anxiety disorders 50
  skills 85
semantic pragmatic language
    disorder 16
separation see parenting
    breakdown
serotonergic antidepressants 133
  anxiety and panic attacks 134
  depression management 24,
      131–2
  learning disabilities 143
serotonergic syndrome 131–2
sertindole, contraindications 130
sertraline 133
  learning disabilities
      treatment 143
sibling rivalry, psychotherapy
    indications 69
single parent families, adolescent
    depression 61
skill acquisition **15**
  critical period 15
sleeper effect 4
sleep problems
  drug treatment 125–6
  learning disabilities 141
social competence programmes 193
social context, cognitive behavioural
    therapy 51
social inclusion, education 187
social perspective taking 49
social phobia, group cognitive
    behavioural therapy 90
social skills training
  group work 80, 86, 92
  IPT-A 57
social support 56
sodium valproate 139
  hypomania/bipolar disorder
      treatment 130

solution focused therapy 115
somatising disorders 173–4
  case example 179–80
  drug treatment 135
special educational needs assessment
    189–92, **190**
specialist referral 18
  indications *25*, 25–6
spectrum disorders, identification
    15–16
statements, special educational
    needs 189
"status tic" 134
storytelling
  family therapy 115
  psychodynamic group therapy 103
strategic family therapy 114
Strengths and Difficulties
    Questionnaire (SDQ) 8
stress
  acute, psychological problems in
    174–5
  interpersonal 97
structural family therapy 114
substance misuse
  confidentiality issues 200
  family therapy 119
sulpiride
  schizophrenia/hallucination
    treatment 127
  tics and Tourette syndrome
    treatment 133
supervision orders 220
supervision strategies 40
"Sure Start" programme 42,
    164–5
surveillance, psychiatric disorders
    13, **13**
symptoms, psychiatric disorders
    12, *12*
systemic therapy 115
systems therapy 20

tardive akathisia, neuroleptic
    induced *128*, 129
tardive dyskinesia, neuroleptic
    induced *128*, 129
tardive dystonia, neuroleptic
    induced *128*, 129

teachers, paediatric wards 195
teasing, psychodynamic group
    therapy 107–8
temperament, role in
    aetiology 7, 8
terminal illness, psychotherapy
    indications 69
tetrabenazine 129, 134
therapists
  cognitive behavioural
    therapy 46, 84
  IPT-A role 56–7
"think aloud" programme 82, **82**
thioridazine, contraindications 130
tics 137
  drug treatment 133–4
topiramate 139
Tourette syndrome, drug treatment
    129, 133–4
tranquillisers 127–30
transitional space, psychodynamic
    group therapy 104
treatment
  context management 19,
    19, 33
  contracts, IPT-A 60
  definitions 19–21
  effectiveness 23–5
  pharmacological medication *see*
    drug treatment
  referral criteria 25–6
  refusal
    case example 206, 209
    guidelines for good practice on
      consent *208–9*
    legal aspects 208–9
    principles 206–8
  settings and staff 21–3
  types 18–27, *19*
  see also individual treatments
trichotillomania, drug
    treatment 133
tricyclic antidepressants
  anxiety and panic attacks 134
  chronic pain management 135
  depression management
    131, 132
  head injury-associated behavioural
    problems 139